New Developments in Home Care Services for the Elderly: Innovations in Policy, Program, and Practice

ALL HAWORTH BOOKS AND JOURNALS
ARE PRINTED ON CERTIFIED
ACID-FREE PAPER

New Developments in Home Care Services for the Elderly: Innovations in Policy, Program, and Practice

Lenard W. Kaye, DSW
Editor

HV
1461
.N47
1995

The Haworth Press, Inc.
New York · London

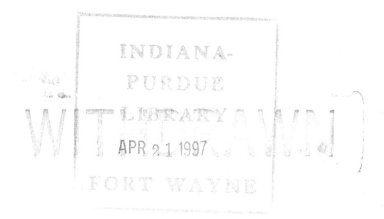

INDIANA-
PURDUE
LIBRARY
APR 21 1997
FORT WAYNE

New Developments in Home Care Services for the Elderly: Innovations in Policy, Program, and Practice has also been published as *Journal of Gerontological Social Work*, Volume 24, Numbers 3/4 1995.

© 1995 by The Haworth Press, Inc. All rights reserved. No part of this work may be reproduced or utilized in any form or by any means, electronic or mechanical, including photocopying, microfilm and recording, or by any information storage and retrieval system, without permission in writing from the publisher. Printed in the United States of America.

The development, preparation, and publication of this work has been undertaken with great care. However, the publisher, employees, editors, and agents of The Haworth Press and all imprints of The Haworth Press, Inc., including The Haworth Medical Press and Pharmaceutical Products Press, are not responsible for any errors contained herein or for consequences that may ensue from use of materials or information contained in this work. Opinions expressed by the author(s) are not necessarily those of The Haworth Press, Inc.

The Haworth Press, Inc., 10 Alice Street, Binghamton, NY 13904-1580 USA

Library of Congress Cataloging-in-Publication Data

New developments in home care services for the elderly : innovations in policy, program, and practice / Lenard W. Kaye, editor.
    p. cm.
Includes bibliographical references and index.
ISBN 1-56024-794-0 (alk. paper)
    1. Aged–Home care–United States. 2. Home care services–United States. I. Kaye, Lenard W.
HV 1461.N47 1995
362.6'3–dc20   95-48902
                                                CIP

FTW
AHY5 310

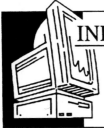# INDEXING & ABSTRACTING

Contributions to this publication are selectively indexed or abstracted in print, electronic, online, or CD-ROM version(s) of the reference tools and information services listed below. This list is current as of the copyright date of this publication. See the end of this section for additional notes.

- *Abstracts in Social Gerontology: Current Literature on Aging*, National Council on the Aging, Library, 409 Third Street SW, 2nd Floor, Washington, DC 20024

- *Academic Abstracts/CD-ROM*, EBSCO Publishing, P.O. Box 2250, Peabody, MA 01960-7250

- *Academic Search: data base of 2,000 selected academic serials, updated monthly: EBSCO Publishing, 83 Pine Street, Peabody, MA 01960*, EBSCO Publishing, 83 Pine Street, Peabody, MA 01960

- *AgeInfo CD-Rom*, Centre for Policy on Ageing, 25-31 Ironmonger Row, London EC1V 3QP, England

- *AgeLine Database*, American Association of Retired Persons, 601 E Street, NW, Washington, DC 20049

- *Alzheimer's Disease Education & Referral Center (ADEAR)*, Combined Health Information Database (CHID), P.O. Box 8250, Silver Springs, MD 20907-8250

- *Applied Social Sciences Index & Abstracts (ASSIA) (Online: ASSI via Data-Star) (CDRom: ASSIA Plus)*, Bowker-Saur Limited, Maypole House, Maypole Road, East Grinstead, West Sussex RH19 1HH, England

- *Behavioral Medicine Abstracts*, University of Washington, School of Social Work, Seattle, WA 98195

(continued)

- *Biosciences Information Service of Biological Abstracts (BIOSIS)*, Biosciences Information Service, 2100 Arch Street, Philadelphia, PA 19103-1399

- *Brown University Geriatric Research Application Digest "Abstracts Section"*, Brown University, Center for Gerontology & Health Care Research, c/o Box G-B 235, Providence, RI 02912

- *caredata CD: the social and community care database*, National Institute for Social Work, 5 Tavistock Place, London WC1H 9SS, England

- *CINAHL (Cumulative Index to Nursing & Allied Health Literature), in print, also on CD-ROM from CD PLUS, EBSCO, and SilverPlatter, and online from CDP Online (formerly BRS), Data-Star, and PaperChase. (Support materials include Subject Heading List, Database Search Guide, and instructional video.)*, CINAHL Information Systems, P.O. Box 871/1509 Wilson Terrace, Glendale, CA 91209-0871

- *CNPIEC Reference Guide: Chinese National Directory of Foreign Periodicals*, P.O. Box 88, Beijing, People's Republic of China

- *Criminal Justice Abstracts*, Willow Tree Press, 15 Washington Street, 4th Floor, Newark, NJ 07102

- *Current Contents. . . . see: Institute for Scientific Information*

- *Expanded Academic Index*, Information Access Company, 362 Lakeside Drive, Forest City, CA 94404

- *Family Violence & Sexual Assault Bulletin*, Family Violence & Sexual Assault Institute, 1310 Clinic Drive, Tyler, TX 75701

- *Human Resources Abstracts (HRA)*, Sage Publications, Inc., 2455 Teller Road, Newbury Park, CA 91320

(continued)

- *Index to Periodical Articles Related to Law*, University of Texas, 727 East 26th Street, Austin, TX 78705

- *INFO-SOUTH Abstracts: contemporary social, political, and economic information on Latin America; available on-line*, North-South Center Consortium, University of Miami, Miami, FL 33124

- *Institute for Scientific Information*, 3501 Market Street, Philadelphia, PA 19104. Coverage in:
  a) Research Alert (current awareness service)
  b) Social SciSearch (magnetic tape)
  c) Current Contents/Social & Behavioral Sciences (weekly current awareness service)

- *Inventory of Marriage and Family Literature (online and CD/ROM), Peters Technology Transfer, Media, PA 19063*, Peters Technology Transfer, 306 East Baltimore Pike, 2nd Floor, Media, PA 19063

- *MasterFILE: updated database from EBSCO Publishing, 83 Pine Street, Peabody, MA 01960*, EBSCO Publishing, 83 Pine Street, Peabody, MA 01960

- *National Clearinghouse for Primary Care Information (NCPCI)*, 8201 Greensboro Drive, Suite 600, McLean, VA 22102

- *New Literature on Old Age*, Centre for Policy on Ageing, 25-31 Ironmonger Row, London EC1V 3QP, England

- *Periodical Abstracts, Research I (general & basic reference indexing & abstracting data-base from University Microfilms International (UMI), 300 North Zeeb Road, P.O. Box 1346, Ann Arbor, MI 48106-1346)*, UMI Data Courier, P.O. Box 32770, Louisville, KY 40232-2770

(continued)

- *Periodical Abstracts, Research II (broad coverage indexing & abstracting data-base from University Microfilms International (UMI), 300 North Zeeb Road, P.O. Box 1346, Ann Arbor, MI 48106-1346)*, UMI Data Courier, P.O. Box 32770, Louisville, KY 40232-2770

- *Psychological Abstracts (PsycINFO)*, American Psychological Association, P.O. Box 91600, Washington, DC 20090-1600

- *Social Planning/Policy & Development Abstracts (SOPODA)*, Sociological Abstracts, Inc., P.O. Box 22206, San Diego, CA 92192-0206

- *Social Science Citation Index. . . . see: Institute for Scientific Information*

- *Social Science Source: coverage of 400 journals in the social sciences area; updated monthly; EBSCO Publishing, 83 Pine Street, Peabody, MA 01960*, EBSCO Publishing, P.O. Box 2250, Peabody, MA 01960-7250

- *Social Sciences Index (from Volume 1 & continuing)*, The H.W. Wilson Company, 950 University Avenue, Bronx, NY 10452

- *Social Work Abstracts*, National Association of Social Workers, 750 First Street NW, 8th Floor, Washington, DC 20002

- *Sociological Abstracts (SA)*, Sociological Abstracts, Inc., P.O. Box 22206, San Diego, CA 92192-0206

(continued)

SPECIAL BIBLIOGRAPHIC NOTES

related to special journal issues (separates)
and indexing/abstracting

☐ indexing/abstracting services in this list will also cover material in any "separate" that is co-published simultaneously with Haworth's special thematic journal issue or DocuSerial. Indexing/abstracting usually covers material at the article/chapter level.

☐ monographic co-editions are intended for either non-subscribers or libraries which intend to purchase a second copy for their circulating collections.

☐ monographic co-editions are reported to all jobbers/wholesalers/approval plans. The source journal is listed as the "series" to assist the prevention of duplicate purchasing in the same manner utilized for books-in-series.

☐ to facilitate user/access services all indexing/abstracting services are encouraged to utilize the co-indexing entry note indicated at the bottom of the first page of each article/chapter/contribution.

☐ this is intended to assist a library user of any reference tool (whether print, electronic, online, or CD-ROM) to locate the monographic version if the library has purchased this version but not a subscription to the source journal.

☐ individual articles/chapters in any Haworth publication are also available through the Haworth Document Delivery Services (HDDS).

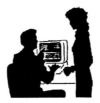

ABOUT THE EDITOR

Lenard W. Kaye, DSW, is Professor at Bryn Mawr College Graduate School of Social Work and Social Research in Bryn Mawr, Pennsylvania. He received his bachelor's degree from the State University of New York at Binghamton, his master's degree from New York University School of Social Work, and his doctorate from the Columbia University School of Social Work. He is the author of *Home Health Care* (Sage Publications, 1992), the coauthor of *Resolving Grievances in the Nursing Home* (Columbia University Press, 1984), and *Men as Caregivers to the Elderly* (Lexington Books, 1990), and the coeditor of *Congregate Housing for the Elderly* (The Haworth Press, Inc., 1991). His forthcoming books include *Controversies in Aging* (Allyn & Bacon), *Part-Time Employment for the Lower Income Elderly: Experiences from the Field* (Garland Publishing), *Self-Help Support Groups for Older Women* (Taylor and Francis), and *Elderly Men: Problems and Potential* (Springer Publishing). He has published approximately 100 journal articles and book chapters on issues in elder caregiving, long-term care advocacy, home health and adult day care, marketing techniques in the human services, retirement life styles, and social work curriculum development.

Dr. Kaye sits on the editorial board of the *Journal of Gerontological Social Work*. He is a board member of numerous community organizations, the Past President of the New York State Society on Aging and of Understanding Aging, Inc., and a Fellow of the Gerontological Society of America. He has recently conducted research with the support of the AARP Andrus Foundation on self-help support groups for older women and on the delivery of high technology home health care services to older adults.

New Developments in Home Care Services for the Elderly: Innovations in Policy, Program, and Practice

CONTENTS

About the Contributors

Miriam K. Aronson, EdD, is Director of the Institute on Aging at Bergen Pines County Hospital, a multiservice campus with 1200 beds, in Paramus, New Jersey, and Associate Professor of Preventive Medicine and Community Health, New Jersey Medical School. A social gerontologist, Dr. Aronson is interested in several important issues facing our aging society, including: correlates of successful aging; risk factors for developing a dementing illness; care of demented individuals and their caregivers; and improving health services. A founder of the National Alzheimer's Association, Dr. Aronson is a member of various local, state and national committees related to aging and health services including membership on the Ethics Committee of the Valley Home Health Care Agency. She has published three books and numerous articles in peer-reviewed journals. Dr. Aronson has extensive case management experience as a private geriatric care manager.

Ann Burack-Weiss, DSW, is Adjunct Associate Professor at the Columbia University School of Social Work. She is engaged in agency consultation, in-service training, and participates nationally in workshops and seminars to advance practitioner skills. A 1989 recipient of the Social Worker in Aging Award of the New York City Chapter of the National Association of Social Workers, Dr. Burack-Weiss is co-author of three books as well as sole author of several papers and book chapters in the professional literature.

Carole Cox, DSW, is Associate Professor in the School of Social Service, The Catholic University of America in Washington, DC. She is author of *The Frail Elderly: Problems, Needs, and Community Responses* (Auburn, 1993) and co-author (with A. Monk) of *Home Care for the Elderly: An International Perspective* (Auburn House, 1991). She is presently conducting research on services for

© 1995 by The Haworth Press, Inc. All rights reserved. *xiii*

Alzheimer's families and hospice care for AIDS patients. Dr. Cox has contributed many chapters and articles on gerontology to various books and journals.

Joan K. Davitt received her masters' degrees from Bryn Mawr College Graduate School of Social Work and Social Research. She holds two degrees, Master of Social Service and Master of Law and Social Policy. Ms. Davitt has worked in gerontology for over 10 years and has conducted research in elder abuse and neglect, housing options for older adults, advance directives in long-term care, and high-tech home health care for older adults. Ms. Davitt has given numerous presentations on long-term care issues to national, state and local groups, as well as to a variety of home care providers. She is co-editor of *A Guide to Nursing Homes in Philadelphia* and has published several journal articles and manuals.

Joanne Handy is Assistant Director, University of California, San Francisco/Mount Zion Medical Center and Executive Director of the Mount Zion Institute on Aging. Her career in home care spans eighteen years as a staff nurse, clinical nurse specialist, supervisor and administrator. She is a past-President of the California Association for Health Services at Home and the recipient of its highest honor, the Lois Lillick Award. Ms. Handy currently serves on the Boards of the National Association for Home Care and the American Society on Aging. She is a Fellow in the prestigious Kellogg International Leadership Program, focusing on home and community-based care.

Susan L. Hughes, DSW, directs the Program of Research in Long Term Care at the Center for Health Services and Policy Research of Northwestern University. She is also Professor in the Department of Preventive Medicine in the Medical School at Northwestern and an Associate Research Career Scientist at the Hines V.A. Hospital Center for Cooperative Studies in Health Services. She has been Principal Investigator of several nationally significant studies of community-based long term care. She has authored numerous articles on community-based long term care as well as the critically acclaimed text, *Long Term Care: Options in an Expanding Market.* She currently serves on the Editorial Board of *Health Services*

Research and is Chair of the Gerontological Health Section of the American Public Health Association.

Marshall B. Kapp, JD, MPH, was educated at Johns Hopkins (BA 1971), George Washington (JD With Honors 1974), and Harvard (MPH 1978). He is a Professor in the Departments of Community Health and Psychiatry and Director, Office of Geriatric Medicine & Gerontology, Wright State University School of Medicine, Dayton, OH. He is also a member of the adjunct faculty at the University of Dayton School of Law. Kapp is a Fellow of the Gerontological Society of America.

Lenard W. Kaye, DSW, is Professor at the Graduate School of Social Work and Social Research at Bryn Mawr College. He has conducted research and published widely on topics in nursing home advocacy and ombudspersons, adult day care, elder caregiving, retirement lifestyles, and curriculum development in administration, program development, and information systems. His research on marketing techniques in gerontological programming and high-tech home health care was supported by grants from the AARP Andrus Foundation.

Toba Schwaber Kerson, Professor in the Graduate School of Social Work and Social Research at Bryn Mawr College is the author of: *Medical Social Work: The Pre-Professional Paradox; Understanding Chronic Illness: The Medical and Psychosocial Dimensions of Nine Diseases; Social Work in Health Settings;* and *Field Instruction in Social Work Settings*. She presently serves on the editorial boards of *Journal of Women & Aging* and *Arete* and is the Book Review Editor of *Social Work in Health Care*. Professor Kerson holds a Doctorate in Social Work and a PhD in Sociology from the University of Pennsylvania.

Renee W. Michelsen, MSS, LCSW, is Director of Elder Care Services at Morristown Memorial Hospital. Ms. Michelsen is the author of "Social Work Practice with the Elderly: A Multifaceted Placement Experience" and "Hospital Based Care Management for the Frail Elderly," and holds a Master of Social Service degree from the Graduate School of Social Work and Social Research, Bryn

Mawr College. She serves on many community boards and committees helping to meet the service needs of and creating new and innovative partnerships for the frail elderly, has been a direct practitioner, administrator, and program planner, and has been a caregiver for several elderly relatives.

Abraham Monk, PhD, is Professor of Social Work and Gerontology at the Columbia University School of Social Work in New York City and Director of the Institute on Aging at Columbia University. He is the author and editor of numerous books and more than 100 journal articles and book chapters in the fields of aging, social planning, and evaluative research. Dr. Monk has conducted extensive research on intergenerational relations, elder housing, long-term care, pre-retirement preparation and post-retirement adjustment, and policy formation concerning families of the aged. He has also conducted past research of home care services in six countries, with a grant from the USDHHS-Administration on Aging.

Janet Neff, RN, BSN, is a Registered Nurse for Baylor HomeCare in Dallas, Texas. She is currently the MIS Educator. She has been in charge of all training on their current information system and is involved in developing RFP's and further selection/training for future clinical systems.

Joan Quinn, RN, MSN, is president of Connecticut Community Care, Inc., and Community Care Network of Connecticut, Inc., as well as The National Case Management Partnership. She also serves as Secretary for Connecticut Long-Term Care Research, Inc. She was the Executive Director of Triage, Inc., a nationally recognized community-based health research and demonstration program. She is recognized for her expertise in long-term care case management. Ms. Quinn is the author of numerous publications, most recently a book entitled *Successful Case Management in Long-Term Care,* and is the founder and editor of the *Journal of Case Management.* She is an advisory committee member regarding case management issues for the United States Office of Technology Assessment, the General Accounting Office, and the Assistant Secretary for Planning and Evaluation of the United States Department of Health and Human Services.

Karen Roberts, MSSW, is the supervisor for social work with Baylor HomeCare, Dallas, Texas. She is a Ph.D. student, teaching assistant, and field placement instructor at the University of Texas at Arlington School of Social Work.

Lucy Rosengarten, ACSW, is founder and executive manager of COHME, Inc. Her background includes ten years as a geriatric social worker in a hospital-based home care program, a year studying cooperative home care management in Bologna, Italy, and training and certification as a home health aide. Ms. Rosengarten, a member of the social work faculty at Mount Sinai Medical School, has taught case management in a variety of community settings and has published in professional journals.

Ellen P. Rosenzweig, is an attorney and the Co-Director of the Institute on Law and Rights of Older Adults, Brookdale Center on Aging of Hunter College, City University of New York (the Law Institute) in New York City. After being in private practice for nine years specializing in estate and trust law, she became a staff attorney at the Institute of Law, an inter-disciplinary resource center which specializes in providing benefit and entitlement information through training of and publications for attorneys, social workers, health care administrators, and other professionals working with the elderly. At the Law Institute, she has specialized in Medicaid, protective services, and home care and participated actively in home care advocacy groups and advisory councils at the City and State levels. She graduated from Brooklyn Law School.

Dick Schoech, PhD, is Professor at the University of Texas at Arlington School of Social Work. He teaches administrative and community practice and computer applications. He is currently on contract with the Texas Department of Protective and Regularity Services to Develop multimedia based tests, training, and employee performance support systems.

Joanne Kennedy Shiffman, RNC, GNP, a Certified Geriatric Nurse Practitioner, received her Masters of Science in Nursing from Seton Hall University. She is presently a member of the Geriatric Evaluation and Management team at the Institute on Aging, Bergen

Pines County Hospital in Paramus, New Jersey. Mrs. Shiffman has been a R.N. for the past eighteen years, working with and teaching disabled and elderly populations in acute, rehabilitation and home care settings.

Preface

It is a pleasure to publish this extraordinary collection of papers. Lenard W. Kaye, a member of the Editorial Board of *Journal of Gerontological Social Work*; and Professor at the Graduate School of Social Work and Social Research at Bryn Mawr College, is the Editor of this Volume and the author of the Introduction, which merits a careful read, and of a chapter on marketing. It is a tribute to Professor Kaye's standing in the field and his perseverance that he was able to engage such an array of leading scholars and policy and program analysts.

This look at *New Developments in Home Care Services for the Elderly* could not be more timely, given the emphasis in Washington and in state capitols across the nation, on home care. Alas, this emphasis is often viewed as a cost containment strategy, rather than valued, as it should be, as a central provision in the system of long-term care and as the provision which is most congruent with the preferences of functionally dependent older people and their families.

I recommend this volume to the readers, and to their colleagues in gerontology and geriatrics. It is a magnificent collection, and, I believe, a real addition to the literature of the field and the profession.

Rose Dobrof, DSW

[Haworth co-indexing entry note]: "Preface." Dobrof, Rose. Co-published simultaneously in *Journal of Gerontological Social Work* (The Haworth Press, Inc.) Vol. 24, No. 3/4, 1995, p. xxi; and: *New Developments in Home Care Services for the Elderly: Innovations in Policy, Program, and Practice* (ed: Lenard W. Kaye) The Haworth Press, Inc., 1995, p. xix. Single or multiple copies of this article are available from The Haworth Document Delivery Service [1-800-342-9678, 9:00 a.m. - 5:00 p.m. (EST)].

© 1995 by The Haworth Press, Inc. All rights reserved.

Introduction

Lenard W. Kaye, DSW

THE PROLIFERATION OF HOME CARE PROGRAMS

Amidst the growing concern that the chronic state of federal resource scarcity will do harm to the scope and breadth of programs for older persons and other vulnerable populations, in-home services have managed to thrive. In fact, the number of organizations providing home-delivered attendant, homemaker, home health aide, nursing, social work, and therapy services is growing at a feverish pace.

The National Association for Home Care identified a total of 15,027 home care agencies in the United States as of March 1994 (National Association for Home Care, 1994). This tally includes Medicare-certified home health agencies, Medicare-certified hospices, and other agencies that do not participate in Medicare. There are probably thousands of additional programs beyond those recognized by the National Association of Home Care that are scattered throughout the country providing low-tech social support, friendly visiting, escort, shopping, and chore services.

While still representing a relatively limited segment of the health care sector, with a growth rate of between 15 to 20% per year, home care is the fastest growing component of the health care delivery system (Handy, 1994). Whether one conceives of in-home services as including the delivery of technology-enhanced, medically intensive services, hospice care, social support, long-term maintenance

[Haworth co-indexing entry note]: "Introduction." Kaye, Lenard W. Co-published simultaneously in *Journal of Gerontological Social Work* (The Haworth Press, Inc.) Vol. 24, No. 3/4, 1995, pp. 1-6; and: *New Developments in Home Care Services for the Elderly: Innovations in Policy, Program, and Practice* (ed: Lenard W. Kaye) The Haworth Press, Inc., 1995, pp. 1-6. Single or multiple copies of this article are available from The Haworth Document Delivery Service [1-800-342-9678, 9:00 a.m. - 5:00 p.m. (EST)].

© 1995 by The Haworth Press, Inc. All rights reserved.

and custodial care, or periodic friendly visiting and reassurance, more and more communities can lay claim to having such services available to their citizens. Estimates of total home care spending from all sources (Medicare, Medicaid, private insurance, out-of-pocket, and other) in 1994 ranged from $23.7 to $29.9 billion or roughly 3% of national health care spending (National Association for Home Care, 1994).

Eighty-six percent of the respondents to an informal survey of home health agencies, visiting nurse associations, home medical equipment and respiratory companies, infusion providers, and hospices recently indicated that they expected to expand their businesses in the next two years (*Home Health Line*, 1994). Furthermore, not-for-profit, voluntary, and public programs providing home attendant, case management, homemaker, and related services commonly report that their agencies have extended waiting lists made up of applicants requesting various forms of assistance in their homes.

Not only is there growing demand for in-home services and greater numbers of home care agencies in our communities, but there is also an increasingly wide range of organizational sponsors and auspices of such programs. Hospitals, nursing homes and other acute and chronic care institutions are now increasingly likely to offer home care services in addition to their more traditional, in-house services. Sectarian and nonsectarian agencies, for-profit and not-for-profit organizations, public and voluntary agencies, and even relatives and friends of the elderly as independent contractors of publicly financed in-home care, are all counted among the current cadre of providers of home care interventions of one kind or another. Publicly-held, multi-unit proprietary chains, often providing low-tech forms of care, are, in particular, fast becoming common features of the home care landscape (Hughes, 1992; Kane, 1989).

THE CALL FOR QUALITY CARE

Amidst the expansion of home care services can be heard the call that such programs operate in a responsible manner. Because the government is paying more for home care, through Medicare and

Medicaid funding streams primarily and through the Older Americans Act and state social service block grants secondarily, one can expect heightened governmental expectations that such services be sound and quality assured (Kramer, Shaughnessy, Bauman, and Crisler, 1990; Balinsky, 1994; Kane, 1994). The rapidly expanding managed-care environment is also being accompanied by additional expectations that home care and other health care providers deliver superior service. Consumer advocacy groups and the public are voicing similar concerns. Yet, the fact that home care exists in so many shapes and forms leads to questions about the capacity of such providers to deliver home care services in a consistent manner reflecting high levels of effectiveness and efficiency.

THE RATIONALE FOR THIS SPECIAL VOLUME

This collection of readings aims to respond to the recurring call for quality in home care service provision. Deemed relevant for home care programs of varying type, scope, and breadth, it presents to agency administrators, managers, supervisors, and front line service providers a set of the most up-to-date policy, program, and practice developments in the field. Offering this collection of readings is premised on the belief that home care agencies need individually-tailored, organizational, managerial, and supervisory guidelines, that are prescriptive in nature and broadly applicable.

This volume is also premised on the appreciation that while home care agencies provide services to persons of all ages, their primary consumers are, more likely than not, older adults. Indeed, home care has taken on an undeniable gerontological focus (Kaye and Davitt, 1994). A large proportion of service beneficiaries are already 75 years of age or older; and, home care recipients of the future are likely to be an increasingly aged cohort. Age is and will remain an important predictor of the need for home care services. Thus, the emphasis in this volume is on the special needs of home care agencies serving older patient populations. Nevertheless, it should be noted that the practice principles and innovation found within will often be transferable with considerable application value to agencies serving younger, functionally impaired persons.

DIVERSITY AND HOME CARE

Given the substantial diversity characterizing the field, home care services are, necessarily, defined broadly for the purposes of this volume. The continuum of home care is seen to include: house-keeping services; escort services; personal care services; case management services; self-care education, teaching, and training services; social-therapeutic services; nursing/medically related services; rehabilitative services; and durable medical equipment (Kaye, 1992). This complex continuum of care assumes necessarily the involvement of a wide range of paraprofessional and professional staff. The involvement of diverse staff extends to all levels of program operation including: administration, management, supervision, and direct service provision. Consequently, the presentations in this volume were conceived to be of immediate relevance to a multidisciplinary audience having both direct service (field) and indirect service (office) responsibilities in the home care organization. Social workers, nurses, business administrators, and public health professionals should find the discussions to be germane in particular.

Above all else, this collection speaks to an appreciation for the increasing organizational and interventive complexity of home care. Home care is perceived to have all the hallmarks of a full-fledged programmatic specialty in the health and human services. This primer responds to the need for a specialized set of principles of practice to inform those engaged in the home care enterprise both today and into the future.

THE CHARGE GIVEN
TO THE VOLUME'S CONTRIBUTORS

The multidisciplinary group of contributors to the volume were chosen based on their capacity to contribute specialized analyses of emergent policy, program, and practice innovation impacting on the organization and delivery of home health care services to older adults and other persons confined to their homes. A range of current topics in the organization and delivery of human services generally, and home care services specifically, are addressed with special attention given to a consideration of the implications of each issue/innovation for: (a) home care agency administration; (b) multidisciplinary home care staffing; and (c) direct service to elderly clients and their families.

Contributors, depending on their areas of acknowledged expertise, were asked to draw on their own applied research and/or professional experience and apply it to the field of home health care. Each was charged with the responsibility for exploring issues of client/staff diversity and the challenges associated with working with clients grappling with various disabling conditions. Specific topics addressed in this collection include:

- home care entitlements and benefits;
- legal and ethical issues in home health care;
- alternative organizational models in home care;
- the importation of high technology services into the home;
- information systems and the field of home care;
- evaluating and monitoring the effectiveness of in-home care;
- marketing home health care services;
- counseling the homebound client and his/her family;
- supervisory challenges for the home care worker;
- clinical assessment tools and packages in home health care;
- case management and the home care client; and
- home care service experiences in other countries.

Taken together, these topics serve to highlight the organizational and service delivery challenges confronting home care providers as they position themselves to meet the challenges of serving growing numbers of persons who need assistance to maintain themselves in their homes.

ACKNOWLEDGMENTS

Appreciation is extended to Rose Dobrof for encouraging the compilation of this volume. Sincere thanks is extended to the contributors to this work as well. Their expertise and breadth of knowledge are most impressive. Their cooperative spirit and prompt response to editorial remarks was most appreciated. They are, of course, responsible for making this volume as strong a document as it is.

REFERENCES

Balinsky, W. (1994). *Home care: Current problems and future solutions.* San Francisco, CA: Jossey-Bass.

Handy, J. (1994). "Challenges and innovations." In Handy, J. and Schuerman, C.K. (Eds.). *Challenges and innovations in homecare.* San Francisco, CA: American Society on Aging.

Home Health Line. (1994). "Home care marketplace: Most providers report business up, plan to expand–not sell," *Home Health Line,* XIX, 6-7.

Hughes, S.L. (1992). "Home care: Where we are and where we need to go." In Ory, M.G. and Duncker, A.P. (Eds.). In *In-home care for older people: Health and supportives services.* Newbury Park, CA: Sage Publications.

Kane, M. (1989). "The home care crisis of the nineties," *The Gerontologist,* 22, 24-31.

Kane, R.A. (1994). "Approaches to quality assurance in homecare." In Handy, J. and Schuerman, C.K. (Eds.). *Challenges and innovations in homecare.* San Francisco, CA: American Society on Aging.

Kaye, L.W. (1992). *Home health care.* Newbury Park, CA: Sage Publications.

Kaye, L.W. and Davitt, J.K. (1994). *High-tech home health care: An analysis of service delivery and consumption.* Bryn Mawr, PA: Bryn Mawr College.

Kramer, A.M., Shaughnessy, P.W., Bauman, M.K., and Crisler, K.S. (1990). "Assessing and assuring the quality of home health care: A conceptual framework," *The Milbank Quarterly,* 68, 413-440.

National Association for Home Care. (1994). *Basic statistics about home care 1994.* Washington, DC: National Association for Home Care.

PART I:
POLICY INNOVATION

Chapter 1

Trends in Home Care Entitlements and Benefits

Ellen P. Rosenzweig, JD

Home care services are currently funded through a patchwork of entitlement and benefit programs, none of which were initially designed to systematically provide long term care for chronically disabled individuals. Medicare, the largest public payor for home care, was designed primarily as an acute care benefit. Only through a national class action lawsuit, *Duggan v. Bowen*, was the focus of the Medicare home health benefit changed from acute care to long term care for chronically impaired individuals. Medicaid initially also focused on acute care, and only the skilled home care services are mandated on states. Medicaid does, however, allow states the option of providing the less skilled home care services through optional state plan services and waiver programs (described in detail, see p. 15). Many states have chosen to provide substantial amounts of less skilled home care services through the Medicaid program. The other federal benefits and entitlements for home care services–Social Service Block Grants, Older Americans Act programs and Veterans Administration and Department of Defense programs are underfunded and limited in the scope or duration of benefits they can provide. Finally, states have not been able to

[Haworth co-indexing entry note]: "Trends in Home Care Entitlements and Benefits." Rosenzweig, Ellen P. Co-published simultaneously in *Journal of Gerontological Social Work* (The Haworth Press, Inc.) Vol. 24, No. 3/4, 1995, pp. 9-29; and: *New Developments in Home Care Services for the Elderly: Innovations in Policy, Program, and Practice* (ed: Lenard W. Kaye) The Haworth Press, Inc., 1995, pp. 9-29. Single or multiple copies of this article are available from The Haworth Document Delivery Service [1-800-342-9678, 9:00 a.m. - 5:00 p.m. (EST)].

© 1995 by The Haworth Press, Inc. All rights reserved. *9*

devote much of their own limited general revenue dollars to provide the less skilled home care services which are needed by an increasingly older disabled population.

In 1993, Health Care Financing Administration (HCFA) officials expected that an estimated $33 billion, including public and private funds, would be spent on home and community-based long term care *for all populations* and projected that 32% would be financed from Medicare, 22% from Medicaid and 46% from private sources (Vladek, Miller & Clauser, 1993). The HCFA projection did not give amounts funded by Older Americans Act funds, Social Service Block Grants, Veteran Administration programs, and state general revenue funding, estimated by others to comprise 23% of public funding for home and community-based care *for the elderly* (Feder, 1991).

A recent Administration on Aging survey of state expenditures on home and community-based care which *excludes* Medicare-funded home health care and food subsidies from the Department of Agriculture collected data for the first time on funding sources used by states to provide home and community-based care *to the elderly* (Administration on Aging, 1994). Based on 1992 figures, the survey concludes that $6.4 billion of federal and state funding, exclusive of Medicare was used to pay for home and community-based services for the elderly. The AoA study figures show that nationally, exclusive of Medicare, states' funding of home care is attributable 69.4% to Medicaid, 10.2% to Social Service Block Grants, 7.8% to Older Americans Act funds, 10.9% to general state revenues and 1.8% to other sources.

These percentages vary dramatically, however, from state to state, as does the amount spent on services per capita of persons age 65 and above. Maine, for example, uses 82.5% from Medicaid, 0% from Social Service Block Grants, 4.2% from Older Americans Act funds and 13.3% of general state revenues to provide $189 of home care services per capita for persons over age 65. California, providing $240 of services per capita for persons age 65 and above, uses 44.5% of Medicaid, 48.35% Social Services Block Grant funds, 6.5% Older Americans Act funds, .5% general state revenues and .2% other funds. New York provides the highest amount of home care services at $1,180 per capita for persons age 65 and above,

96% from Medicaid funds. Mississippi, providing the least amount of home care funding at $29 per capita for persons age 65 and above, uses 15.2% from Medicaid funds, 45.5% from Social Services Block Grant funds, 30.3% from Older Americans Act funds and 0% from state revenues and other sources. These state variations indicate the flexibility which states currently have in using different levels of funding from various federal sources to design their programs but also demonstrate that, without a coherent federal funding stream, states are free to provide extremely limited amounts of home care services in addition to those covered by Medicare.

The figures also demonstrate that exclusive of Medicare, Medicaid is the only federal program providing significant funding of home care services. Oregon, the second highest funder of home care at $369 per capita for persons age 65 and above, uses 89.7% from Medicaid; California, the next highest at $240 per capita for persons age 65 and over, uses 44.5% from Medicaid; and Washington at $212 per capita for persons age 65 and over, uses 62% from Medicaid (Administration on Aging, 1994).

A substantial amount of the cost of home care is still paid out-of-pocket by the elderly. Estimates of average out-of-pocket long term home care spending by both the elderly and the disabled projected by the Brookings Institution over the 1991-1995 period constituted 37.6% of the total projected cost (Weiner, Ilston and Hanley, 1994b). Private long term care insurance currently pays for only one percent of *total* long term care expenses (Weiner et al., 1994b), most of which presumably covers nursing home care rather than home care.

In addition to private spending for home care services, a large but unmeasured amount of the services used by the elderly and disabled at home is provided informally by family and friends. In 1989, only an estimated 29% of the disabled elderly at home were using paid home care services (Weiner et al., 1994b). Approximately 4.2 million spouses and adult children of disabled elderly persons living at home provide assistance with activities of daily living and another three million relatives, friends or neighbors also are actively providing informal care (Stone, 1991). In fact, most elderly and disabled individuals would be unable to remain at home even with paid home care without the supervision and assistance of an informal caregiver. The importance of informal care is now well recognized as is the importance of providing services such as adult day care and respite care to support informal caregivers.

This chapter will discuss each of the public sources of funding available for home care services for the elderly and disabled, describe, briefly, developments in private long term care insurance coverage of home care and present some of the trends in home care financing currently under development.

MEDICARE

Use of the Medicare home health entitlement has grown substantially since 1980. This increase is attributable to the removal of the three day prior hospitalization requirement and the 100 visit limit in 1980, the adoption in 1983 of the prospective payment system for hospital benefits which reduced the length of stay for hospital visits thus shifting care previously provided in hospital to home settings and the 1989 changes in Medicare home health coverage after the *Duggan v. Bowen* lawsuit which expanded the home health benefit from an acute care focus to more of a long term care benefit for chronically impaired individuals (Leader, 1991; Bishop and Skwara, 1993). Spending for Medicare home health benefits increased at an annual average rate of 40% between 1988 and 1991 as a result of the *Duggan* revisions in the coverage guidelines (Bishop, 1993). Predictably, the rapid increase in Medicare home health expenditures has prompted an internal HCFA review to improve, among other things, the efficiency, accountability and fiscal integrity of the program (HCFA, 1994). Whether an attempt to limit the benefit will result remains to be seen.

Medicare covers primarily skilled medical home health services–part-time or intermittent nursing, physical, speech and occupational therapy and home health aide. Private duty nursing is not covered. Personal care services (assistance with activities of daily living) are funded by Medicare only to the extent that they are "incidental" to medical home health services and are not covered as a stand-alone service. Social work services are covered if they are needed to insure the effectiveness of medical treatment.

Medicare coverage is divided into two parts, Part A (hospital insurance) and Part B (medical insurance). Part A covers home health services, but persons enrolled only in Part B are covered for the same home health services under the same eligibility requirements as Part A enrollees.

Medicare home health eligibility rules are set forth in detail in the *Medicare Health Insurance Manual* (HCFA pub. 11), known as the H.I.M. 11. Note that the kinds and amounts of services covered are not set forth in statute or regulation, but rather are detailed in HCFA prepared manuals. The home health manual provisions were rewritten at the conclusion of the *Duggan v. Bowen* law suit. The Medicare home health eligibility rules are complicated and consist of three sets of criteria which the individual must meet to receive services: the qualifying criteria, the coverage criteria and the reasonable and necessary criteria.

There are five qualifying criteria, all of which must be met to qualify for Medicare coverage of home health care. First, a physician must certify the need for the services and must draw up and periodically review the treatment plan. Second, the individual must remain under the care of a physician. Third, the care must be intermittent skilled nursing care (defined as either less than 5 days a week but at least once every 60 days or daily for a finite and predictable amount of time) *or* physical therapy, *or* speech therapy *or* continuing occupational therapy after physical therapy has terminated. Fourth, the individual must be "homebound," defined as unable to leave the home because of illness or injury without the assistance of a person or device and without a considerable and taxing effort (trips from the home for medical reasons or short and infrequent trips for non-medical purposes are acceptable if all of the other requirements of the definition are met). Fifth, the home health agency providing services must be certified by Medicare.

If all five of the above qualifying criteria are met, Medicare will pay for the kinds and amounts of home health services, defined in the coverage criteria, provided the services are medically reasonable and necessary. Combined skilled nursing and home health aide services are covered if they are part-time (defined as seven days a week and less than eight hours per day and up to a maximum of 28 hours [or 35 hours if additional documentation supports the extra hours] per week for an indefinite period of time) *or* intermittent (defined as either less than seven days a week and up to 28 [or 35 with additional documentation] hours per week for an indefinite period of time or seven days a week, eight hours a day, for a finite and predictable period of time). Note that home health aide services are not covered unless the skilled nursing or therapy qualifying criteria are met. Physical therapy, speech therapy, occupational therapy, medical social work and medical supplies and equipment are also covered. Medicare does not cover full-time nursing care, drugs (except immunosuppressive drugs) or meals delivered to the home. Homemaker, chore services or personal care services are *not* covered unless *incidental* to patient care which is being provided by a home health aide.

Finally, even if the qualifying and coverage criteria are met, the services must still be "medically reasonable and necessary." Prior to the revision of the H.I.M. 11, Medicare denials were often couched in terms of lack of medical necessity. The revised Manual clarified that a finding that services are not medically reasonable and necessary must be based upon information provided in the plan of care and the medical record with respect to the unique medical condition of the individual. In addition, the Manual provides that determinations of whether care is "skilled" must be made without regard to whether the illness or injury is acute, chronic, terminal or expected to extend over a long period of time.

Note that, since 1980, a three day prior hospitalization is *not required* for Medicare coverage of home health care as it is for Medicare covered nursing home care. Currently, Medicare pays for home health services in full; that is, without a deductible or co-payment. Many of the recent health care reform and budget proposals, however, considered by Congress impose co-payments on Medicare home health.

A Medicare determination of eligibility is initially made by the Medicare certified home health agency. This determination is not appealable by the individual applicant unless the applicant demands that the home health agency submit the claim for services to Medicare despite the agency's good faith belief that the services will not be covered. If Medicare denies coverage, the applicant will then have to pay privately for the services received, but will also have gained the right to appeal the Medicare coverage denial. Many Medicare home health care denials are reversed on appeal.

Medicare will pay for hospice services from a Medicare-approved hospice once a doctor certifies that the patient has only about six months to live. The hospice philosophy of terminal care requires that patients choose to forego active treatment and receive only palliative care. Those patients who choose hospice receive a combination of home and institutional services, although hospice is primarily a home care program and most hospice patients die at home. Home care services include home health aide and personal care services, at least one weekly visit from a registered nurse, medical equipment and supplies, drugs, support for family members involved in caregiving and occasional respite. Although hospice has generally been used to provide care to terminally ill cancer patients, about 10% of patients have illnesses other than cancer, the most common being cardiac diagnoses and chronic lung disease (Scanlon, 1994). An increased use of the hospice benefit for terminal care can be anticipated as the population reaching advanced old age continues to grow.

MEDICAID

Unlike Medicare, which is funded entirely by the federal government, Medicaid is a joint federal and state program, funded half by the federal government and half by the states. In contrast to Medicare, an insurance program which covers most elderly and disabled individuals without regard to their income and resources, Medicaid is designed to cover certain categories of individuals with very low income and resources. Federal legislation and regulation set forth the general requirements which states must follow, making coverage of some categories of individuals and some benefits mandatory and some optional.

The Medicaid categorical and financial eligibility rules are beyond the scope of this discussion, except to state that blind, elderly and disabled recipients of Supplemental Security Income (SSI) cash assistance are required to be covered in all states unless the state opts to use more restrictive definitions of blindness or disability or use more restrictive eligibility standards than SSI as long as the standards are no more restrictive than the Medicaid eligibility rules in effect in that state on January 1, 1972. Twelve states currently use this option (Connecticut, Hawaii, Illinois, Indiana, Minnesota, Missouri, New Hampshire, North Carolina, North Dakota, Ohio, Oklahoma and Virginia). In all other states, SSI recipients must be covered by Medicaid. Beyond that, states may provide services to other optional classes of people such as the elderly, blind and disabled who have income and resources above the Supplemental Security Income level and those with medical bills which reduce their income level to the state's Medicaid income level. States vary greatly in their categorical and financial eligibility criteria, and expert advice should be obtained to determine whether an individual is financially and categorically eligible in a particular state.

In addition to deciding which groups of state residents are categorically and financially eligible, states also have great flexibility in choosing which services to cover under their Medicaid programs. Federal law and regulation set forth minimum required or mandated benefits and allow states the option of providing other services. States may provide home care services under three provisions of the federal Medicaid statute: state plan home health services; state plan optional services such as personal care services, private duty nursing, respiratory therapy and hospice; and so-called "waiver" programs.

Mandatory and optional services offered under the Medicaid state plan in a particular state must meet certain federal requirements–the services must be uniformly offered throughout the state; the recipient must have free choice of providers; comparable services must be available to all individuals within the mandated groups and within each of the other groups covered by the state; and any limits placed on the amount of services must be "sufficient in amount, duration, and scope to achieve the purposes of the Medicaid program." If states wish to provide services without complying with these state plan requirements, they may obtain a "waiver" of one or more of them under certain federal provisions which allow states to operate programs for special populations, for demonstration programs or for individuals eligible for nursing homes who can be maintained at less cost in the community.

State Plan Home Health Services

Certain home health services are mandatory and others are optional. The mandatory home health services are part-time or intermittent nursing, home health aide and medical equipment and supplies. Optional home health services are physical therapy, occupational therapy, speech pathology and audiology. Most states cover the optional home health services of physical, speech and occupational therapy (Folkemer, 1994). States must cover the mandatory services for all individuals covered for nursing facility services under their Medicaid program. Thus, states such as Alabama and Delaware offer the mandated home health services only to those individuals receiving SSI cash assistance (Miller, 1992; Folkemer, 1994).

In addition, although particular home health services are required in all states, the *amount* of such services is not set by federal law except that a non-waivered service must be of sufficient amount, duration, and scope to achieve the purposes of the Medicaid program. Thus, states which wish to provide the minimum amount of home care may provide only token amounts of the mandated home health services to SSI cash assistance recipients without violating state plan requirements. Alabama, for example, which provides only the mandated home health services to SSI recipients, limits the amount of the mandated services to 104 visits per year (Folkemer, 1994, Fatoullah, 1992). Delaware, the other state which provides only the mandated home health services to SSI recipients, limits the cost of the mandated services to the cost of nursing facility services (Folkemer, 1994, Fatoullah, 1992). At the other end of the spectrum, New York provides both the mandatory and optional home health benefits to all categories of individuals allowed to be covered under the federal Medicaid law without a visit or cost limit, although recent state legislation has sought to impose a cost limitation equal to the cost of nursing home services.

State Plan Optional Services

States may provide optional services at home or in other non-institutional settings under their state plans, subject to the federal requirements of statewideness, provider choice, comparability of services within categories of recipients and sufficient duration in scope. As states have faced increasing budget shortfalls, they have been unwilling to expand optional services because fulfilling the state plan requirements increases the cost of offering these services. The optional home care services which states may offer under their state plans are personal care services, home and community-based care for functionally disabled elderly individuals, private duty nursing, and respiratory therapy for ventilator dependent individuals who otherwise would require institutionalization and hospice.

State Plan Optional Personal Care Services

Personal care services must be prescribed by the person's physician or, at state option, otherwise authorized in accordance with a service plan approved by the state. Personal care services are designed to maintain a frail elderly or disabled person at home and include housekeeping, cleaning, cooking, dishwashing, shopping, laundry, paying bills, physical care such as bathing, grooming, turning, dressing, feeding, and help with transferring, walking, toileting, routine skin care and assistance with taking medication. Thirty-two states provide optional personal care services (Folkemer, 1994).

State Plan Optional Home and Community-Based Care Services for Functionally Disabled Elderly Individuals

Effective July 1, 1991, another optional home care service (known as the "frail elderly" or Section 4711 option) for Medicaid eligible individuals age 65 or over who are unable to perform two of three activities of daily living–toileting, transferring and eating–or who have Alzheimer's disease and meet certain functional disability tests was added. Only one state, Texas, is currently providing services under this option. Rhode Island has received approval, but is not yet operating its program (Folkemer, 1994). States already providing optional personal care or home and community-based waiver services to the elderly have been reluctant to provide this relatively new optional service (Lipson and Laudicina, 1991).

State Plan Optional Private Duty Nursing

States may cover private duty nursing provided by a registered nurse or a licensed practical nurse under the direction of the recipient's doctor in the recipient's home for individuals who require more continuous care than is available from a visiting nurse. "At home" was clarified in 1990 to include private duty nursing outside of the home during those hours when the recipient's normal life activities, such as school or employment, occur outside the home. These locations may be covered only if the individual would have been covered at home during that time period. Twenty-seven states provide the private duty nursing optional benefit (Commerce Clearing House, Inc., 1994). Most states, however, limit the private duty nursing benefit by requiring prior approval or capping hours or cost.

State Plan Optional Respiratory Therapy for Ventilator Dependent Individuals Who Otherwise Require Institutionalization

Respiratory care services may be provided on a part-time basis in the individual's home by a respiratory therapist or other health care professional with appropriate training approved by the state provided that the patient is medically dependent on a ventilator for at least six hours per day, has been so dependent for at least thirty consecutive days (or less days authorized by the state) as an inpatient in a hospital or nursing facility, would continue to require inpatient services unless respiratory care services are available at home, has adequate social support services at home, wishes to be cared for at home and these services are not otherwise available under the state's Medicaid program. Sixteen states provide the optional respiratory therapy service (Commerce Clearing House, Inc., 1994).

State Plan Optional Hospice

The hospice benefit described under the Medicare provisions above can also be covered under Medicaid at state option. Thirty-five states provide the optional hospice program.

Waiver Home Care Programs

States may cover certain other home and community-based services under special provisions of federal law which allow the federal government to "waive" certain Medicaid state plan requirements for states that propose a program of home and community-based services for persons who would otherwise be institutionalized. These services, known as "waivered services," can include case management services, homemaker services, home health aide services, personal care services, adult day health services, rehabilitation services, respite care services, day treatment or other partial hospitalization services, psychosocial rehabilitation and clinic services for persons with chronic mental illness and other services requested by a state which are approved as cost efficient (Commerce Clearing House, Inc., 1994). Some of the other services which states have covered in their waiver programs for the elderly include medical social work services, home maintenance tasks, housing improvements, transportation, congregate/home delivered meals, respite care, emergency response services, moving assistance, respiratory therapy, nutrition counseling/education services, assisted living, adult foster care, mental health services, counseling, etc. (Folkemer, 1994).

Home and community-based waiver programs are available to states under two alternative provisions of federal Medicaid law referred to by the section numbers of the statute–1915(c) and 1915(d). The 1915(c) waivers are limited to chronically ill and disabled persons who would require institutional care without the services offered under the waiver and are not limited to the elderly. States must prove in their 1915(c) waiver application that the cost of the home and community-based services will not be greater than the cost of institutional services would have been for the persons served under the waiver. The formula used to determine these costs has been based on the number of available Medicaid certified beds in the state as well as the projected number of beds to be built and those closed as a direct result of the waiver. This formula resulted in a limit on the number of slots available in a particular state and controlled the growth of 1915(c) waiver programs. Recently proposed federal regulations would simplify this formula and make it easier for states to cover larger numbers of eligible persons. Despite the complexity of the 1915(c) waiver application process, 45 states had 1915(c) waiver programs serving the elderly as of July, 1993. States without such waivers serving the elderly are Arizona, District of Columbia, Oklahoma, Oregon, Pennsylvania and Texas (Folk-emer, 1994).

The 1915(d) waivers authorize home and community-based waivers for persons aged 65 and over who would be placed in a nursing home without the waiver program. The major difference between the 1915(c) and (d) programs is the method of calculating the cost efficiency of the program. Oregon is the only state which has a 1915(d) waiver program.

Although many states have home and community-based waiver programs, these programs need not serve an entire state's geographical area and may target specific populations within a state. For these reasons, the number of individuals served in a particular state's waiver programs is usually small compared to the total population needing such services. States which elect the state plan personal care option serve much greater numbers of eligible persons because of the state plan requirements. Many states have both a personal care program and one or more waiver programs.

SOCIAL SERVICE BLOCK GRANTS

The Social Security Act was amended in 1981 to provide federal funds known as Social Service Block Grants (SSBGs), consolidating all federal assistance to states for social services into a single grant. Each state was directed to furnish services aimed at reducing economic dependency, preventing or remedying neglect, abuse or exploitation of children and adults, reuniting families, preventing or reducing inappropriate institutional placement and providing services to individuals in institutions where appropriate. No federal requirements, other than the general purposes stated above, are placed on the expenditure of these funds, and the use of these funds is not limited to the elderly, blind or disabled.

The funding level for Social Service Block Grants has been capped at the 1981 level of $3 billion nationally and appropriations have remained at around $2.5 billion since then (Brown, 1990). In 1992, the appropriation was $2.8 billion. Of this amount, only $.66 billion was spent on home care for the elderly (Administration on Aging, 1994).

Because states are not required to submit post expenditure reports, little data are available about the kinds of services and populations served by states under the program (Brown, 1990). A state survey, based on 1992 figures, found that some portion of SSBG funds were allotted to home and community-based services for the elderly in 39 states (Administration on Aging, 1994). The kinds of activities that states used SSBGs to fund were homemaker/home health (74%), adult protective (45%) and case management/access (43%) (Brown, 1990). Other activities funded by some states were family assistance, transportation, nutrition/meals, socialization and disabled/handicapped services (Brown, 1990).

OLDER AMERICANS ACT FUNDS

Limited funds are available to states for home and community-based services under Older Americans Act funding, administered through the state units on aging. In 1992, not counting home-delivered meals, about $.5 billion of Older Americans Act funds were spent on in-home services for the elderly (Howard, 1991; Administration on Aging, 1994). Because of the "skimpy" funding (Binstock, 1991) available, the Administration on Aging has had limited success in pursuing one of its major goals, the coordination of community-based systems of care for older adults. Although some state and area agencies on aging have been able to cooperate with other agencies and funding sources to expand and coordinate services, anecdotal evidence suggests that coordinated, comprehensive community-based care has not been developed in most states (Fortinsky, 1991). Nevertheless, the area agency on aging remains the starting point in the search for home and community-based services for older adults and their families in most states and continues to serve as a central repository of information about available services.

BENEFITS FOR VETERANS AND THEIR DEPENDENTS

Despite recent attempts to improve home care services under Veterans Administration (VA) and Department of Defense (DOD) programs, the VA and DOD cover very limited amounts of home care services, leaving elderly veterans, members of the uniformed services and their dependents to rely on Medicare and Medicaid for most of their home care needs. The VA provides direct health care services through VA owned, staffed and operated medical facilities to veterans discharged other than dishonorably. In addition, the VA administers a health insurance program using private sector providers for spouses, unmarried children or survivors of veterans with permanent total disability resulting from service-connected disabilities under the Civilian Health and Medical Program of the Department of Veteran's Affairs (CHAMPVA). The Department of Defense also operates a direct care system and a health benefits program for active duty members, their dependents, retired members, their dependents and survivors of deceased retired and active members of the uniformed services (Army, Navy, Marines, Air Force, Coast Guard, Public Health Services and National Oceanic and Atmospheric Administration). The Civilian Health and Medical Program for the Uniformed Services (CHAMPUS) operates like a private health insurance system.

The VA direct care program provides limited hospital-based home care within short distances from a VA hospital. This program does not cover home health aide or personal care, but provides doctor visits, rehabilitation, social services, dietetic consultations and psychological assessments, prescriptions and durable medical equipment. Unfortunately, the number of veterans served by this program is extremely limited. In 1992, less than half of the VA hospitals provided hospital-based home care, and the average daily census for the program was 5,136 patients (General Accounting Office, 1993). In addition to the direct provision of hospital-based home care services, veterans may receive additional funds to help pay for privately hired home care assistance if they require the regular aid and attendance of another individual to care for them. The VA use of direct cash payments to allow veterans to purchase additional assistance directly is the only federal program currently using this approach. CHAMPVA covers skilled nursing, therapy services, home health aide services, medical equipment and supplies at home. CHAMPUS covers the same services but does not include home health aides. CHAMPUS eligible persons must transfer completely to Medicare if eligible; CHAMPVA eligible individuals can use CHAMPVA benefits to supplement Medicare benefits.

STATE-FUNDED PROGRAMS

Because of the rigid eligibility requirements in the various federal programs discussed above, states have in recent years begun to experiment with programs funded entirely from state revenues. Because of state budget pressures, however, the amount of funding for these programs has been limited. In 1992, $.7 billion was spent nationally from state general revenues, in addition to the state matching funds in the Medicaid program, for home and community-based services (Administration on Aging, 1994). Florida, Illinois, Massachusetts, Minnesota, Pennsylvania and Rhode Island all used state revenues as major funding for community-based programs, often because they felt that costs could be contained more effectively and programs made more flexible outside the constraints of the Medicare and Medicaid programs.

Typically, the financial eligibility requirements for state programs have been set at a higher income level than Medicaid and have employed a sliding cost sharing schedule in order to reach individuals slightly above the Medicaid levels. These cost sharing programs typically do not require that recipients spend down resources to establish eligibility. The services provided are usually the less medical services such as homemaker or chore services, home maintenance and repairs, respite, social day care, etc., often not covered by Medicare at all and not available under Medicaid in those states which do not provide the optional Medicaid personal care benefit and have limited waiver programs. Another strategy often employed in programs funded by state revenues is the use of independent case management to locate services, perform assessments, develop care plans and ensure cost effectiveness of service provision. Many states separate the case management function from the service provision function to make sure that clients receive unbiased recommendations and to avoid conflicts of interest in service authorization (Justice, 1990).

PRIVATE INSURANCE

In the absence of any substantial public coverage of long term costs other than Medicare and Medicaid, a private long term care insurance market has begun to develop, but few elderly have purchased private long term care insurance. Although Medicare covers 97% of the elderly and two-thirds supplement Medicare with private Medicare supplemental policies, perhaps 4-5% of the elderly and a negligible percentage of the non-elderly have purchased some kind of private long term care insurance (Weiner et al., 1994b).

Most state insurance departments have now established minimum standards and some consumer protections for long term care policies. Initially, these policies were often limited to coverage of nursing home expenses, but have now come to include home care as well. A few policies also include adult day care and respite care. Almost all long term care policies are purchased individually by the elderly who must bear the entire cost of the premiums unless younger family members wish to contribute. Affordability is a major concern since premiums are typically expensive. Several studies have found that only between 10-20% of the elderly can currently afford good quality policies with adequate coverage (Weiner, 1994b).

According to recent simulations at the Brookings Institution, private long term care insurance will remain as an option available primarily to upper-income elderly and will have almost no impact on Medicaid expenditures unless the non-elderly, through employer sponsored group policies can be convinced to buy policies (Weiner et al., 1994b). Inflation protection and length of coverage are important features if younger consumers are to be persuaded to purchase long term care policies. Employer sponsored plans are becoming more common and can usually be purchased for the employee's spouse and parents (Boyd, 1990). Whether younger workers, concerned with child care, mortgage payments and college education for their children will actually purchase long term care insurance remains to be seen (Weiner et al., 1994b).

In addition to the growth of the private long term care insurance market, the Robert Wood Johnson Foundation has encouraged states to combine private long term care insurance with Medicaid. Demonstration programs are now under way in Connecticut, New York, California and Indiana which allow individuals to purchase state approved private long term care insurance and then, after using up the insurance benefits, to become eligible for Medicaid without spending down their remaining assets. Iowa, Illinois and Maryland are also considering such projects. Federal legislation passed in 1993, however, prevents expansion of these programs to any other states.

FUTURE ISSUES IN HOME CARE

Although the elderly and disabled clearly prefer to remain at home for as long as possible, many questions remain unresolved in the development of a comprehensive long term care program, not the least of which is how to control home care expenditures (Weiner and Illston, 1994a). Recently, interest in integrating the delivery and funding of acute and long term care has led to various model demonstration projects (Weiner and Illston, 1994a; National Academy for State Health Policy, 1994). In addition, increasingly, advocates for the disabled and the elderly are joining together to discuss the possibilities for a single community-based long term care program which can adequately serve both populations (Weiner and Illston, 1994a).

Without sufficient uniform funding available throughout the states for chronic care services at home, large numbers of the frail elderly and disabled and their caregivers will have to continue to pay privately for home care and rely on friends and family for assistance. For those without funds or informal caregivers to assist them, many will continue to go without needed services or be forced unnecessarily into institutions. Provision of a coherent, adequately funded, home and community based delivery system remains one of the greatest challenges before our society today.

REFERENCES

Administration on Aging. (1994). *Infrastructure of home and community based services for the functionally impaired elderly: State source book.* Washington, DC: Administration on Aging.

American Association of Retired Persons. (1992). "Public policy fact sheet: Home and community-based long-term care." Washington, DC: American Association of Retired Persons.

Ansak, M. (1990). "The On Lok model: Consolidating care and financing," *Generations 14,* 73-74.

Binstock, R.H. (1991). "From the great society to the aging society–25 years of the Older Americans Act." *Generations, 15,* 11-18.

Bishop, C. and Skwara, K.C. (1993). "Recent growth of Medicare home health." *Health Affairs, 12,* 95-110.

Boyd, B. (1990). "LTC insurance: It's your choice." *Generations, 14,* 23-27.

Brown, H.W. (1990). *A survey of the states on the Title XX social services block grant program and services to the elderly.* Washington, DC: American Association of Retired Persons.

Butler, R.N. and Davis, K. (1991). "Forward." In Rowland, D. and Lyons, B. (Eds.). *Financing Home Care: Improving Protection for Disabled Elderly People.* Baltimore, MD: The Johns Hopkins University Press.

Clark, W.D. and Rhodes, R.S. (1994). "State reforms in long term care: Budgets, waivers, and state initiatives as catalysts." *Journal of Long-Term Home Health Care, 13,* 17-28.

Commerce Clearing House, Inc. (1994). *Medicare and Medicaid Guide.* Chicago, IL: Commerce Clearance House, Inc.

Estes, C.L., Swan, J.H. and Associates. (1993). *The long term care crisis: Elders trapped in the no-care zone.* Newbury Park, CA: Sage Publications, Inc.

Fatoullah, E. (1992). "Medicaid home care for the elderly and persons with disabilities." *Clearinghouse Review, 26,* 882-897.

Feder, J. (1991). "Paying for home care: The limits of current programs." In Rowland, D. and Lyons, B. (Eds.). *Financing Home Care: Improving Protection for Disabled Elderly People.* Baltimore, MD: The Johns Hopkins University Press.

Folkemer, D. (1994). *State use of home & community-based services for the aged under Medicaid: Waiver programs, personal care, frail elderly services and home health services.* Washington, DC: American Association of Retired Persons.

Fortinsky, R.H. (1991). "Coordinated, comprehensive community care & the Older Americans Act." *Generations, 15,* 39-42.

General Accounting Office. (1993). Comparison of VA benefits with other public and private programs. GAO/HRD-93-94. Washington, DC: U.S. Government Printing Office.

General Accounting Office. (1994). *Medicaid long-term care: Successful state efforts to expand home services while limiting costs.* GAO/HEHS-94-167. Washington, DC: U.S. Government Printing Office.

Harrington, C. and Newcomer, R.J. (1990). "Social health maintenance organizations as innovative models to control costs." *Generations, 15,* 49-54.

Health Care Financing Administration. (1994). Issue paper: The Medicare home health initiative (for discussion purposes only). Washington, DC: Health Care Financing Administration.

Howard, E.F. (1991). "Long-term care: On the comeback trail?" *Generations, 15,* 39-42.

Justice, D. (1990). "State community-based care systems: Striking a balance between flexibility & cost control." *Generations, 14,* 45-48.

Leader, S. (1991). "Medicare's home health benefit: Eligibility, utilization, and expenditures." *Issue Brief: A Monthly Publication from the Public Policy Institute of AARP*, No.1. Washington, DC: American Association of Retired Persons.

Leutz, W.N., Greenlick, M.R., and Capitman, J.A. (1994). "Integrating acute and long-term care." *Health Affairs, 13*, 58-74.

Lewis-Idema, D., Falik, M., and Ginsberg, S. (1991) "Medicaid personal care programs." In Rowland, D. and Lyons, B. (Eds.). *Financing home care: Improving protection for disabled elderly people.* Baltimore, MD: The Johns Hopkins University Press.

Lipson, L. and Laudicina, S. (1991). *State home and community-based services for the aged under Medicaid: Waiver programs, optional services under the Medicaid state plan, and OBRA 1990 provisions for a new optional benefit.* Washington, DC: American Association of Retired Persons.

McCarthy, M.E. (1994). *VA manual.* Carson City, NV: Nevada Legal Services, Inc.

Miller, N.A. (1992). "Medicaid 2176 home and community-based waivers: The first ten years." *Health Affairs, 11*, 162-171.

National Academy for State Health Policy and American Association of Retired Persons. (1994). *Integrating acute and long-term care: Advancing the health care reform agenda, Conference proceedings.* Washington, DC: American Association of Retired Persons.

National Association for Home Care. (1994). "Basic Statistics About Home Care." Washington, DC: National Association for Home Care.

Neuschler, E. (1991). "Medicaid eligibility for frail elders." In Rowland, D. and Lyons, B. (Eds.). *Financing Home Care: Improving Protection for Disabled Elderly People.* Baltimore, MD: The Johns Hopkins University Press.

Perkins, J., Melden, M., and Regan, M. (1993). *An advocate's guide to the Medicaid program.* Los Angeles, CA: National Health Law Program.

Regan, J.J. (1990). "Home care and the government: Regulations and reimbursement." In Zuckerman, C., Dubler, N.N. and Collopy, B. (Eds.). *Home Health Care Options: A Guide for Older Persons and Concerned Families.* New York, NY: Plenum Press.

Rowland, D. and Lyons, B. (1991). "The elderly population in need of home care." In Rowland, D. and Lyons, B. (Eds.). *Financing Home Care: Improving Protection for Disabled Elderly People.* Baltimore, MD: The Johns Hopkins University Press.

Rowland, D. and Lyons, B. (1991). "A proposal to expand home care benefits." In Rowland, D. and Lyons, B. (Eds.). *Financing Home Care: Improving Protection for Disabled Elderly People.* Baltimore, MD: The Johns Hopkins University Press.

Scanlon, B.C. (1994). "Hospice for aged persons without cancer: The experience of the Hampshire County (MA) hospice." *Journal of Long-Term Home Health Care, 13*, 37-45.

Stone, R. (1991). "Familial obligation: Issues for the 1990s." *Generations, 15,* 47-50.

Vladek, B.C., Miller, N.A., and Clauser, S.B. (1993). "The changing face of long term care." *Health Care Financing Review, 14,* 5-23.

Weiner, J.M. and Hanley, R.J. (1992). "Caring for the disabled elderly: There's no place like home." In Shortell, S. and Reinhardt, U. (Eds.). *Improving Health Policy and Management: Nine Critical Research Issues for the 1990s.* Ann Arbor, MI: Health Administration Press.

Weiner, J.M. and Illston, L.H. (1994a). "Health care reform in the 1990s: Where does long-term care fit in?" *The Gerontologist, 34,* 402-408.

Weiner, J.M., Illston, L.H., and Hanley, R.J. (1994b). *Sharing the Burden: Strategies for Public and Private Long-Term Care Insurance.* Washington, DC: The Brookings Institution.

Chapter 2

Legal and Ethical Issues in Home-Based Care

Marshall B. Kapp, JD, MPH

There is a strong and growing emphasis in the United States on providing long term care services both formally (i.e., by paid agencies and professional personnel) and informally (i.e., by family members or friends) to mentally and physically disabled individuals, primarily but not exclusively the elderly, in their own home environments. Both formal and informal home caregiving for disabled persons engender a rich and inescapable array of legal and ethical considerations for the various professionals and lay persons engaged in this enterprise. The most salient of these issues are outlined in this chapter.

REGULATORY FRAMEWORK

Home care delivery takes place within a context of extensive federal and state regulation (Kapp, 1992a, pp. 183-189). The vast majority of states currently require the licensure of home care agencies, whether proprietary or not-for-profit, as a precondition of operation. Promulgated under the state's inherent *police power* authority, these licensure statutes are intended to promote and protect

[Haworth co-indexing entry note]: "Legal and Ethical Issues in Home-Based Care." Kapp, Marshall B. Co-published simultaneously in *Journal of Gerontological Social Work* (The Haworth Press, Inc.) Vol. 24, No. 3/4, 1995, pp. 31-45; and: *New Developments in Home Care Services for the Elderly: Innovations in Policy, Program, and Practice* (ed: Lenard W. Kaye) The Haworth Press, Inc., 1995, pp. 31-45. Single or multiple copies of this article are available from The Haworth Document Delivery Service [1-800-342-9678, 9:00 a.m. - 5:00 p.m. (EST)].

© 1995 by The Haworth Press, Inc. All rights reserved.

the health, safety, and welfare of patients. The same rationale under-
lies state statutes in every jurisdiction that regulate members of
individual health care professions (such as physicians, nurses,
psychologists, social workers, and physical and occupational therapists) who may work for a home care agency.

Licensure laws apply regardless of payment source. Home care
agencies participating in the Medicare and Medicaid programs must
also comply with regulatory requirements promulgated by the federal Health Care Financing Administration (HCFA), 56 *Federal
Register* 32967-32975 (July 18, 1991).

In addition to regulation targeted at patient care standards, an
array of federal and state laws impact upon many of the business
aspects of home care delivery. These requirements include, among
others: state health planning and certificate of need laws, Medicare-
Medicaid Antifraud and Abuse provisions, the Sherman Antitrust
Act, and the Robinson-Patman Price Discrimination Act.

Besides these governmental modes of regulation, there exist a
variety of private, voluntary forms of accreditation by nongovern-
mental entities in the home care arena. Although it is not legally
obligatory, there may be strong financial and other incentives for
home care agencies to achieve voluntary accreditation. The main
accreditation bodies here are the Joint Commission on Accreditation of Healthcare Organizations (JCAHO), the National League of
Nursing's Community Health Accreditation Program (CHAP), and
the National Homecaring Council (NHCC).

LEGAL LIABILITY

Relatively few civil malpractice lawsuits have been brought by
or on behalf of patients against home care agencies or individual
home care professionals of any type (American Medical Association, 1991). However, a high anxiety level among home care providers is fanned by a number of social, economic, and technical
factors that may place them at risk, at least theoretically, for potential litigation and liability (Brent, 1989; Haddad & Kapp, 1991,
pp. 171-200; Kapp, 1992a, pp. 189-199).

For one thing, as home care becomes increasingly high-tech for
many patients who previously would have needed institutionaliza-

tion because of the severity of their illnesses or disabilities (Arras and Dubler, in press), the chances for events to go disastrously wrong grow as well. Second, the permeation of home care services with sophisticated technologies, coupled with strong provider financial incentives to keep patients out of acute care hospitals altogether or at least to shorten their lengths of stay as much as possible, often results in a patient demographic picture characterized by a much higher sickness or acuity level than would have been found in the past. Sicker home care patients demanding more complicated and time-consuming kinds of attention increase the potential risk of adverse outcomes, which are a central element of any negligence claim (Erickson & Anderson, 1989).

Although home care patients may be more ill than their predecessors, they and their families usually have higher consumer expectations regarding the availability and quality of their care. These rising expectations apply to patients and families drawn from all racial, ethnic, and gender groups. Additionally, special personnel needs increase the potential liability exposure of home care providers. As the variety and number of personnel required by home care agencies continues to expand (including, for example, R.N.s, L.P.N.s, social workers, occupational therapists, physical therapists, speech therapists, home health aides, and others), so, too, expands the reliance by many home care agencies on purchasing services from independent contractors. Further, the dissemination of home care services to patients through a complex web of sites and individuals presents challenging management information, monitoring, coordination, and supervision difficulties for home care agencies, which can make it more problematic to control legal risks than would be the case if operations were all under one roof (Brueckner and Pace, 1989).

Contractual Liability

One source of possible liability of home care agencies to patients is based on breach or violation of contract. This may occur under several legal theories: (1) violation of express or implied promises to patients made about availability, quality, or price of services contained in the agency's advertising or marketing materials and (2) failure to fulfill promises made directly to patients (or their surrogates), either orally or in the form of written admission and service contracts.

Tort Liability

To date, tort suits (primarily predicated on allegations of negligence or unintentional deviation from acceptable professional standards proximately causing foreseeable injuries) have been relatively rare in the home care sphere. Nevertheless, the perpetual threat of a malpractice action looms as one important legal mechanism for maintaining the quality of services rendered by home care providers and for compensating patients who are negligently harmed (Atkinson, 1987).

Under the theories of personal, vicarious, and corporate liability, an agency and its staff are all amenable to lawsuit for negligence in patient care. Because the agency acts, or fails (omits) to act, only through its staff, the area of selection, assignment, monitoring, and supervision of professional and paraprofessional employees and contractors represents one of the chief liability danger zones in home care.

Another significant negligence risk in the home care setting is the opportunity for patient injury brought about by inadequate communication of relevant information among agency staff or between the home care agency and other providers who are involved in the patient's care. The agency may also be held accountable for negligence in failing to communicate properly with its patients, when patient damage results. The duty to communicate with patients (or their surrogates) includes, among other things, the contexts of informed consent and medication instructions. Effective communication compels home care providers to take into account special barriers or needs occasioned by a patient's particular racial or ethnic background (Randall, 1994).

Products Liability

As noted previously, home care at the end of the twentieth century increasingly entails the use of sophisticated medical equipment. A panoply of problems can happen in this regard (even assuming the equipment has been prescribed properly in the first place) that can engender legal risk in the contingency of patient harm. Product-related risk areas encompass defects in the equipment itself, incorrect installation, improper use by professionals due to insufficient training or to carelessness, and malfunctions caused by patient or family mistakes. In any of these circumstances, the consequences for the patient who depends on the equipment may be dire, and litigation may follow.

For legal purposes, the home care agency is considered to act both as a professional service provider (subject to tort standards of due care) and as the seller of a product (thereby judged according to product liability principles). The agency thus has responsibilities in terms of proper installation, inspection, and supervision of equipment operation, as well as concerning the training of professionals, family, and the patient in the correct use of equipment.

Independent Agencies and Contractors

Home care agencies today rely extensively on independent agencies and practitioners to supply them with certain workers who provide services to patients (Kane, 1989). The primary agency faces potential liability exposure under the doctrines of ostensible or apparent agency and corporate responsibility. Hence, the primary agency is obligated to exercise due care under the circumstances, according to industry standards, in its selection and monitoring of independent contractors. In addition, home care agencies ought to consider negotiating and including in their contracts with outside agencies an indemnification or "hold harmless" clause that prospectively spells out the respective rights and responsibilities of each party in the event of a lawsuit brought by or on behalf of the patient.

Acceptance, Transfer, and Discharge of Patients

A home care agency's legal duties toward a patient grow out of the professional relationship that is formed between the two parties. Hence, the threshold question confronting the agency is whether to enter into a professional relationship with a particular individual in the first place.

An agency, of course, may not discriminate in patient selection according to irrelevant personal attributes such as race, ethnicity, gender, or religion. Beyond that constraint, a home care agency neither should nor may accept a patient unless there is a reasonable expectation that the individual's medical, nursing, and social needs can be met adequately by the agency in the patient's own home. Under the Americans with Disabilities Act (ADA), an agency may not reject an applicant solely on the basis of a disability; rejection is permissible only if the agency would be unable to render adequate quality care to that person. Although a home care agency may place great weight upon the recommendation of a referring physician or facility, it may not legally delegate its duty to perform an adequate assessment and to make the ultimate decision concerning admission of a new patient.

The other side of the coin is determining in which situations a home care agency may transfer or discharge a patient for whom it has been caring. Because individuals might suffer negative physical or emotional reactions (akin to "transfer trauma" in the nursing home context) as a result of such changes in status, care in making and carrying out these decisions is requisite. In terminating a relationship, the agency must be careful to avoid abandoning the patient—that is, leaving the patient who continues to need home care services in the lurch without adequate access to a competent, acceptable source of care. Risk management in this arena suggests developing and implementing a satisfactory discharge planning process (Coleman, 1988).

Miscellaneous Areas

Every state, under its *parens patriae* power to protect vulnerable persons, has enacted statutes dealing with the problem of elder abuse and neglect. A home care agency may be held criminally and civilly liable for severe patient mistreatment committed by its staff. Additionally, agencies must have clear, explicit policies and procedures regarding the detection and reporting by staff of suspected instances of patient abuse and neglect by formal and informal caregivers and other persons in the patient's home. This is a phenomenon that may occur across the patient spectrum.

Another potential source of liability in home care stems from the unauthorized release of sensitive patient-specific information. Agencies must be conversant with the principle of confidentiality and create and implement written protocols for respecting patient privacy and for dealing with exceptions to the general rule (e.g., suspected abuse or neglect, finding of infectious disease) that might arise in the home setting. A patient's particular ethnic heritage may affect expectations about privacy, and providers should be sensitive to this factor.

THE FAMILY'S ROLE

In the home care setting, the patient's family (utilizing that term here in a liberal sense) may be integrated into the caregiving process in two different but quite interconnected ways. The family may be involved in making decisions about specific aspects of the care plan. Particular family members also may function as direct, informal caregivers to the disabled patient. Both of these potential roles carry significant ethical and legal implications.

Decision Making

Family caregivers almost inevitably will be involved in medical decision making concerning disabled relatives for whom they are caring at home, whether or not the patient has the mental capacity to make his or her own decisions. The degree to which this occurs may vary among different racial, religious, and ethnic populations. Many mentally capable persons choose to include their family caregivers extensively in medical decision making. The patient may delegate present or future decision making authority to a specific family member formally, through execution of a durable power of attorney document. Usually, though, the transfer is silent, with the patient superficially acting as decision maker but in reality relying completely on the family caregiver's opinion. Decisionally capable patients may also depend on family members to various lesser extents without totally transferring decision making authority to them. Many cognitively impaired individuals may find it hard to make adequately competent decisions on their own, but may be made capable "enough" with the support and assistance of family caregivers (Pratt, Jones, Shin, and Walker, 1989; Kapp, 1990).

Indeed, for the decisionally capable individual who needs home care and wishes to receive at least some of it informally, family caregiver participation in care plan decisions is pragmatically unavoidable. Even where they are not effectively acting as the decision makers, the agreement and cooperation of family caregivers is an essential source of psychological and practical empowerment, enabling or helping the patient to carry out personal desires. Absent the family caregiver's involvement in this way, any patient preferences requiring that somebody actually "do" something would go unrealized (Kapp, 1992b). The patient's right to select specific courses of action imposes correlative obligations (i.e., obligations to effectuate those decisions) on the part of family caregivers.

From a strict legal perspective, family caregiver involvement in decision making for the mentally *in*capable home care patient is more straightforward. Where the patient presently lacks decisional capacity because of dementia or other cognitive or emotional impairment, ordinarily family caregivers step in as substitute decision makers. The traditional preference for family members as proxies is grounded in a belief that they are most likely to be aware of and guided by the patient's values or, if those values are unknown in a specific situation, most likely to make decisions consistent with the patient's best interests (High, 1988; Doukas, 1991).

Unless the family has been explicitly disempowered (by, for example, the patient appointing a non-relative as agent under a durable power of attorney), formal providers usually look to relatives even in the absence of an express proxy creation instrument such as a durable power of attorney or guardianship order. This traditional practice may be buttressed by the slew of family consent statutes enacted by state legislatures (Minikoff, Sachs, and Siegler, 1992).

Hence, formal home care providers usually rely on family members of decisionally incapable patients without insisting on formal directives or judicial oversight. The family decision making hierarchy is frequently clearer in the home care setting than in many other service delivery sites. Ordinarily, the family member with whom the decisionally incapacitated lives takes on the main responsibility for decision making, and the rest of the family goes along.

Family as Caregivers

The majority of home care in the United States at present is provided informally. Where willing and able family members are available, it is typical for home care agencies or hospital or nursing facility discharge planners to train those relatives (most commonly wives, daughters, and daughters-in-law) to provide certain services (primarily personal care and homemaker services) for the patient. Instruction should be provided in a variety of formats, such as workbooks, checklists, and audiovisual tapes. Documentation of the teaching process and the family caregivers' progress is vital.

Formal providers need to establish a system for adequately monitoring the family's performance and for responding to any adverse alterations in the patient's health status, including problems related to deficiencies in family caregiving. There should be in place a process for continuous feedback to, and improvement of, family caregiving performance. This process must include provisions pertaining to provider response in the extreme and sensitive event of suspicion of abuse or neglect of the patient by a family caregiver (O'Malley, Everitt, O'Malley, and Campion, 1983).

Professional licensure laws may act as a complicating factor concerning informal caregiving by families, especially regarding health-related services such as giving medications and operating medical equipment. Most state Nurse Practice Acts explicitly exempt from their restrictions those services provided by family (and in the majority of cases friends also) to relatives in their own homes. No state explicitly empowers family caregivers to administer medications or other medical treatments; neither do most states expressly prohibit family from doing so. Despite the murkiness of the family caregiver's exact legal status, as a practical matter relatives help home care patients to take medications and use medical machinery thousands of times a day without any legal repercussions for practicing nursing or medicine without a license.

DECISIONS TO LIMIT TREATMENT

Legal and ethical dilemmas about the initiation, continuation, withholding, or withdrawal of life-sustaining medical treatments

(LSMTs) are not restricted to institutional settings. Increasingly, home care providers are confronted with these questions, as end-of-life medical decisions are both made and carried out in the patient's home (Kapp, in press; Haddad and Kapp, 1991, pp. 79-99).

Issues concerning the execution and interpretation of advance medical directives are relevant to home care. Advance directives may be of the instructional (i.e., "Living Will") or proxy (i.e., Durable Power of Attorney) type. The Patient Self-Determination Act (PSDA) passed by Congress as part of the Omnibus Budget Reconciliation Act (OBRA) of 1990 expressly applies to Medicare and Medicaid certified home health agencies (as well as hospitals, nursing facilities, hospices, and the health maintenance organizations and preferred provider organizations through which home care may be obtained) (Haddad, 1994). While this federal statute, Public Law 101-508 §§ 4206 and 4751, and the implementing regulations promulgated by the Department of Health and Human Services (DHHS), 42 C.F.R. § 489.102, are not intended to create new substantive patient rights, they impose several new procedural requirements on covered health care providers.

Specifically, certified home care agencies are mandated to: (1) create written policies and procedures, consistent with state statutory and judicial law, regarding how they will handle advance directives; (2) provide written information to new patients or their surrogates regarding state law on advance directives and the provider's policy on implementing the state law; (3) document whether the patient has executed an advance directive; and (4) offer decisionally capable patients the opportunity to voluntarily execute such a directive. However, no patient may be coerced into taking this action.

Examples of successful experiences with the use of advance medical directives in the home care setting are abundant (Markson and Steel, 1990). Most home care patients have welcomed the initiation of discussions about future treatment preferences (Daly and Sobal, 1992), although one's racial or ethnic background may influence his or her attitudes in this arena (Randall, 1994). When patients subsequently become decisionally incapacitated and seriously ill, both professionals on the interdisciplinary care team and proxy decision makers find their previous discussions with the patient and the patient's documented wishes to be quite helpful in fulfilling the patient's autonomy.

Another kind of advance or prospective medical directive is a physician's order to other members of the care team directing them not to engage in particular interventions for that patient. Such "Do Not" orders could pertain to hospitalization, intubation, or many other potential actions that might be imposed on a patient for purportedly therapeutic reasons. "Do Not" orders emanate from discussions with a presently decisionally capable patient, an incapacitated patient's advance instruction directive, conversations with the earlier competent patient, and/or discussions with family or friends who are functioning as surrogates either under a durable power of attorney, guardianship appointment, family consent statute, or custom.

Most legal and ethical inquiry to date concerning "Do Not" orders has dealt with the specific technology of cardiopulmonary resuscitation (CPR) (American Heart Association, 1992, Part VIII). There exists a well-established legal and ethical presumption in favor of beginning CPR for a patient who has suffered a cardiac arrest. This presumption may be rebutted, however, where the patient and/or family believe that the forseeable burdens of the attempt are likely to outweigh the reasonably expected benefits (Blackhall, 1987; Dull, Graves, Larsen, and Cummins, 1994).

PHYSICAL OR CHEMICAL RESTRAINTS

Family caregivers who are experiencing heavy physical and emotional stress may ask the physician to prescribe, and nurses to implement, psychotropic drugs or mechanical restraints for the patient as a method of behavior management (Post, 1992). The ethical dilemma of the physician and supporting members of the home care management team may be exacerbated by an implied (and sometimes even express) threat that, if medical help to control the patient's behavior is not forthcoming, the family may be left with no choice but to place the patient in an institution.

The home care team surely needs to be sensitive to the family strains associated with home care of disabled persons, especially demented individuals. Nonetheless, physical and chemical restraints usually increase the probability of serious patient injury, as demented persons drugged into stupor struggle to free themselves from restraining devices that often are misapplied by family or formal caregivers initially or inadequately monitored following application. Thus, the legal and ethical presumption must be against restraint use and in favor of at least first trying less intrusive behavior control alternatives.

FACING LEGAL AND ETHICAL CHALLENGES PROACTIVELY

Home care providers from all disciplines confront a panoply of legal and ethical challenges in carrying out their daily activities. The delivery of home care services has become far too complex an enterprise in the 1990s to continuously deal with these issues on an emergency, *ad hoc* basis. To the maximum extent feasible, these challenges should be identified, anticipated, and prepared for in an organized, proactive manner.

A comprehensive, formal risk management program is advisable for home care agencies to implement as a strategy designed to reduce legal (and thus financial) exposure resulting from injuries to patients (Dronsfield, 1990) and others (e.g., reducing staff worker compensation claims). At the least, liability insurance coverage or a sufficiently-funded self-insurance program, as well as staff education, should be included (Brueckner & Pace, 1989; Erickson & Anderson, 1989). Written agency policies and procedures should be created as needed and regularly updated. An occurrence- or incident-reporting and follow-up system is another essential component of risk management (Connaway, 1986).

Another facet of risk management that is especially relevant in the home care arena, where supervision is so spread out and care and supplies may be secured through numerous subcontracts, is a mechanism offering patients and their families the opportunity to provide comments directly to agency management about their feelings concerning the quality of care received. These perceptions, particularly when critical, should then be investigated and responded to by management to preempt or reduce potential problems and to maintain good relations generally with patients and their families. Sensitivity to pertinent racial and ethnic characteristics of patients and families is imperative here.

Ethics committees and/or trained ethics consultants are available to assist home care agencies to foresee and prepare for specifically ethical challenges (Haddad and Kapp, 1991, pp. 208-216). An ethics committee is a formal, multidisciplinary group comprised of representatives from both within and outside an agency who bring to the table a variety of relevant perspectives and areas of expertise. The actual composition, structure, and operation of an ethics committee are matters to be decided upon at the particular agency level. Similarly, the agency must decide which of the following functions its own ethics committee will pursue: policy formulation and review; staff, patient, family, and public education; concurrent case review; and retrospective case review. If an ethics committee is assigned to concurrent case review, it may operate either in an advisory capacity or merely as a forum for the expression of various viewpoints. Virtually no ethics committees are authorized to render binding decisions for an agency or institution, although in a few cases courts have cited ethics committee recommendations in support of upholding the propriety of provider conduct. A home care agency may opt to sponsor its own ethics committee or to pool resources with other agencies in a regional effort.

As a supplement or an alternative to the ethics committee approach, an agency might consider retaining an individual ethics consultant to assist with policy formulation, educational, and case analysis functions as the need is perceived. An agency may also bring in experts to conduct periodic ethics audits evaluating the agency's performance concerning the anticipation and resolution of potential ethical dilemmas.

CONCLUSION

Just as the renewed intensive emphasis on home care represents the cutting edge of long term care in the contemporary United States, the legal and ethical implications of home care exist in a dynamic state. Recognizing, shaping, and responding to these interesting issues in a productive way will both challenge and reward those who plan, administer, and deliver home care services now and into the next century.

REFERENCES

American Heart Association, Emergency Cardiac Care Committee and Subcommittees. (1992). "Guidelines for cardiopulmonary resuscitation and emergency cardiac care: Ethical considerations in resuscitation," *Journal of the American Medical Association, 268,* 2282-2288.

American Medical Association, Council on Scientific Affairs. (1991). "Educating physicians in home health care," *Journal of the American Medical Association, 265,* 769-771.

Arras, J.D. and Dubler, N.N. (Eds.). (In Press). *Bringing the hospital home: Ethical and social implications of high-tech home care.* Baltimore: Johns Hopkins University Press.

Atkinson, S.C. (1987). "Medicare cost containment and home health care: Potential liability for physicians and hospitals," *Georgia Law Review, 21,* 901-927.

Blackhall, L.J. (1987). "Must we always use CPR?" *New England Journal of Medicine, 317,* 1281-1285.

Brent, N.J. (1989). "Risk management in home health care: Focus on patient care liabilities," *Loyola University Law Journal, 20,* 775-795.

Brueckner, G. and Pace, D. (1989). "Implementing an effective home care risk management program," *Perspectives in Healthcare Risk Management, 9,* 25-28.

Coleman, S. (1988). "Discharge planning for the home health agency." In O'Hare, P.A. and Terry, M.A. (Eds.), *Discharge planning: Strategies for assuring continuity of care.* Rockville, MD: Aspen Publishers.

Connaway, N.I. (1986). "Incident reports in home health agencies," *Home Healthcare Nurse, 4,* 9-10.

Daly, M.P. and Sobal, J. (1992). "Advanced directives among patients in a house call program," *Journal of the American Board of Family Practice, 5,* 11-15.

Doukas, D.J. (1991). "Autonomy and beneficence in the family: Describing the family covenant," *Journal of Clinical Ethics, 2,* 145-153.

Dronsfield, J.C. (1990). "Home health services." In Harpster, L.M. and Veach, M.S. (Eds.), *Risk management handbook for health care facilities.* Chicago: American Hospital Publishing.

Dull, S.M., Graves, J.R., Larsen, M.P., and Cummins, R.O. (1994). "Expected death and unwanted resuscitation in the prehospital setting," *Annals of Emergency Medicine, 23,* 997-999.

Erickson, J. and Anderson, M. (1989). "Strategies for managing risk outside the hospital: Home health agencies," *Perspectives in Healthcare Risk Management, 9,* 29-31.

Haddad, A.M. (1994). "The Patient Self-Determination Act in the home care setting." In Kapp, M.B. (Ed.), *Patient self-determination in long-term care: Implementing the PSDA in medical decisions.* New York: Springer Publishing Company.

Haddad, A.M. and Kapp, M.B. (1991). *Ethical and legal issues in home health care.* Norwalk, CT: Appleton & Lange.

High, D.M. (1988). "All in the family: Extended autonomy and expectations in surrogate health care decision making," *Gerontologist* (Supp.), *28*, 46-51.

Kane, N.M. (1989). "The home care crisis of the nineties," *Gerontologist, 29*, 24-31.

Kapp, M.B. (In Press). "Problems and protocols for dying at home in a high tech environment." In Arras, J.D. and Dubler, N.N. (Eds.), *Bringing the hospital home: Ethical and social implications of high-tech home care.* Baltimore: Johns Hopkins University Press.

Kapp, M.B. (1992a). *Geriatrics and the law: Patient rights and professional responsibilities,* 2nd ed. New York: Springer Publishing Company.

Kapp, M.B. (1992b). "Who's the parent here? The family's impact on the autonomy of older persons," *Emory Law Journal, 41*, 773-803.

Kapp, M.B. (1990). "Informed, assisted, delegated consent for elderly patients," *AORN (Association of Operating Room Nurses) Journal, 52*, 857-862.

Markson, L. and Steel, K. (1990). "Using advance directives in the home-care setting," *Generations* (Supp.), *14*, 25-28.

Minikoff, J.A., Sachs, G.A., and Siegler, M. (1992). "Beyond advance directives: Health care surrogate laws," *New England Journal of Medicine, 327*, 1165-1169.

O'Malley, T., Everitt, D., O'Malley, H., and Campion, E. (1983). "Identifying and preventing family-mediated abuse and neglect of elderly persons," *Annals of Internal Medicine, 98*, 998-1005.

Post, S.G. (1992). "Behavior control and Alzheimer disease in perspective," *Alzheimer Disease and Associated Disorders, 6*, 73-76.

Pratt, C.C., Jones, L.L., Shin, H.Y., and Walker, A.J. (1989). "Autonomy and decision making between single older women and their caregiving daughters," *Gerontologist, 29*, 792-797.

Randall, V.R. (1994). "Ethnic Americans, long term care providers, and the Patient Self-Determination Act." In Kapp, M.B. (Ed.), *Patient self-determination in long-term care: Implementing the PSDA in medical decisions.* New York: Springer Publishing Company.

PART II:
PROGRAM INNOVATION

Chapter 3

Alternative Organizational Models in Home Care

Joanne Handy, RN

Organizational structures of home care providers mirror the diversity and complexity of the home care field itself. The business literature commonly describes the home care "industry" in terms of four major segments: (1) home health services, ranging from nursing and therapy to homemaking; (2) hospice care; (3) home medical equipment, including respiratory therapy; and (4) home infusion therapy (Yessne, 1994). Another typology identifies four models of home care in the United States as high-tech home care, hospice, skilled home health care and low-tech custodial care (Hughes, 1992). Within these broad categories, home care is often further subdivided by auspice, such as voluntary or proprietary. When described in terms of services, home care encompasses a potential list of 101 services, which can be delivered as single services, or clustered into groups. These services range from traditional nurses and homemakers to pet care, massage, and grocery delivery (National Association for Home Care, 1992). Such distinctions will increasingly blur as home care providers evolve into integrated home care delivery organizations. For now, this segmentation remains a useful way of describing a complex field.

[Haworth co-indexing entry note]: "Alternative Organizational Models in Home Care." Handy, Joanne. Co-published simultaneously in *Journal of Gerontological Social Work* (The Haworth Press, Inc.) Vol. 24, No. 3/4, 1995, pp. 49-65; and: *New Developments in Home Care Services for the Elderly: Innovations in Policy, Program, and Practice* (ed: Lenard W. Kaye) The Haworth Press, Inc., 1995, pp. 49-65. Single or multiple copies of this article are available from The Haworth Document Delivery Service [1-800-342-9678, 9:00 a.m. - 5:00 p.m. (EST)].

© 1995 by The Haworth Press, Inc. All rights reserved.

This article explores the determinants of organizational structure, discusses organizational success factors, and describes emerging models that reflect the forces impinging on home care providers today. It will focus primarily on the skilled and paraprofessional service sectors of the field, and to a lesser extent, on the product and equipment sectors.

DETERMINANTS OF ORGANIZATIONAL STRUCTURE

If form truly did follow function, the organizational structure of home care services might be simpler than exists today. The form, however, is influenced by myriad factors beyond function. Some of the most influential factors include: strategic focus; corporate structure of the sponsor; licensure, certification and accreditation; and industry norms.

Strategic Focus

Strategic focus is the process of concentrating effort, activity and resources on those particular markets and products that achieve organizational success (Tweed, 1993). Strategic focus operationalizes an organization's mission by defining those customers and services that will achieve the mission. New agencies entering the home care arena, or existing providers adding home care to their current business repertoire, initially determine whether they want to provide skilled home health services (nursing, social work, therapies), personal care and homemaker services, or both; whether they want to provide services on an intermittent or shift basis, (also referred to as per visit or continuous care), or both. This determination significantly defines the administrative models that will be used.

Corporate Status

If home care services are but one of several services offered, the corporate status of the parent entity may determine organizational form. According to the National Association for Home Care

(NAHC), there are 15,027 home care agencies in the United States, 7,521 of whom are Medicare certified home health agencies. Of the Medicare certified providers, 2,892 are for-profit, 2,081 are owned by hospitals, 1,146 are government run, 586 are Visiting Nurse Associations (VNA) and 123 are owned by skilled nursing facilities. Comparable data on noncertified agencies, which comprise the bulk of shift care, personal care and homemaker providers, is not available (National Association for Home Care, 1994).

Until 1994, hospitals and skilled nursing facilities had a distinct financial incentive to organize certified home health agencies as departments of their institutions. Medicare allowed these institution-based providers to include a percentage of their overall administrative and general overhead in calculating their visit costs. The Medicare cost reimbursement system then recognized a higher cost cap for these institutions. In response to federal cost pressures and the urging of other types of home care providers to "level the playing field," the institutional-based add-on was eliminated in 1994.

The corporate configuration often determines the way in which administrative functions are carried out for the home care service. In institution-based and corporate branch organizations, marketing, client billing, and human resource functions are commonly carried out by the hospital or corporate office. This arrangement can lead to economies of scale and the ability to develop a competitive pricing structure, or burden the home care service with high overhead costs, resulting in higher prices.

Licensure/Certification/Accreditation

Depending upon the type of home care service provided, state licensure or Medicare certification may be required, and significantly impacts administrative structure. There are currently thirty-three states that have licensing laws for home care, applicable primarily to agencies providing skilled nursing or personal care services, not to agencies providing only homemaker or attendant services. These licensing requirements, which vary widely from state to state, can be quite prescriptive about governance functions, staffing ratios and supervision of services. For example, California's licensing law at present requires a full-time director of nursing and a supervisory ratio of one supervisor to 12 full-time equivalent nurses for any organization that sends nurses into a person's home (California Administrative Code, 1982).

Home care agencies participating in the Medicare program must also meet the Medicare Conditions of Participation. Like state licensing laws, the conditions specify minimum standards in the areas of agency administration, home care records, policies and procedures, client rights, safety management, and quality assurance.

Accreditation for all types of home care providers is available through the Community Health Accreditation Program (CHAP) of the National League for Nursing and the Joint Commission on Accreditation of Healthcare Organizations (JCAHO). Initially considered the "gold" standard, accreditation is evolving quickly to be an important indicator of overall agency quality and a business necessity. Third party payors and referral sources increasingly require accreditation as a condition of contracts, and efforts to educate consumers about the benefits of accreditation are mounting. The accreditation requirements reflect higher standards than licensing or certification requirements, are more outcome oriented, and have a strong emphasis on continuous quality improvement. Both CHAP and JCAHO also have standards for providers whose main focus is on personal care and support services, including companions, chore service workers, home attendants, personal care aides, homemakers and home health aides. The CHAP has recently been granted "deemed status" under Medicare, meaning that it can certify agencies for Medicare participation in the course of its accreditation process.

Industry Norms

In a rapidly changing business and service environment, organizations modify their internal structures to respond to market forces. Four types of change characterize the home care field: specialization, segmentation, consolidation, and integration. On a broad level, the dominant strategy employed by home care organizations is horizontal or vertical integration. Horizontal integration refers to organizing complimentary or related services within one level of care; e.g., a home care organization that offers skilled services, infusion therapy, medical equipment and homemakers. Vertical integration refers to strategies that link different levels of care; e.g., a health care system that offers primary care, acute care, home care, long term institutional care and community services. On a programmatic level, the trend is toward privatization; i.e., developing service delivery structures outside the Medicare model that has played a pivotal role historically in how services are organized. A common example is providing shift or per visit skilled services for managed care or private insurance clients through a separate division of an agency, utilizing separate staff and delivery systems. In this manner, the higher overhead costs associated with Medicare are avoided, and agencies can be more price competitive in their service.

It has been noted that for-profit organizations are more likely than nonprofit to respond to market forces by changing their organizational structure (Estes, 1988). However, the ability to respond quickly to change may have more to do with the complexity of the organization than its tax status.

Benchmarking is a useful process for comparing one's organization to industry norms. Benchmarking involves the systematic collection of information on key performance parameters from industry-leading organizations, ideally in similar market territories. Information for benchmarking is collected on field staff/supervisor ratios, administrative staff/service staff ratios, productivity requirements for both field and office staff, pay rates, costs and charges per visit. This information is derived from surveys, telephone interviews, review of publicly available agency reports and state and national trade associations.

ORGANIZATIONAL SUCCESS FACTORS

Certain characteristics contribute to success of home care providers as they adapt to the rapidly changing health care environment. A 1993 report prepared by Ernst and Young for the Home Health Assembly of New Jersey identified the following success factors:

1. Clarity of role–Providers will need to focus their resources around major opportunities that exist. This can be providing new services to existing clients; expanding scope along the

service spectrum; i.e., from maintenance home care to high tech services; or shifting functions; i.e., from direct service provider to care management.

2. External market focus–Providers need to thoroughly understand the buyer market, be it government, insurance payors, businesses or consumers themselves.

3. Ability to track costs–Providers will need a detailed understanding of the costs of care by service, by client and by condition in order to assume risk on contracts.

4. Ability to document positive outcomes–Providers will need to document health and functional outcomes of their services, requiring the development of clinical and management information systems.

5. Organizational responsiveness and flexibility–Home care organizations need the ability to quickly reorganize services and personnel to meet the needs of the external marketplace (e.g., forming a dedicated managed care team to care for managed care clients).

6. Ability to negotiate contracts and capitalize on political power–Home care providers need the negotiating skills to develop successful contracts and the relationship building skills that assure their effective participation in networks that are developing (Home Health Assembly of New Jersey, 1993).

EXAMPLES OF ORGANIZATIONAL MODELS

The home care field presents many varieties of organizational models that reflect the determinants described above. Three examples are briefly outlined here to illustrate the types of models that are quite common in the industry.

1. A Horizontally Integrated VNA

The Visiting Nurse Service of Rochester and Monroe County in New York offers an example of a large, multiservice, horizontally integrated organization. As indicated in Chart I, the VNS is comprised of three corporate entities: the Visiting Nurse Foundation,

CHART I. Visiting Nurse Service of Rochester and Monroe County

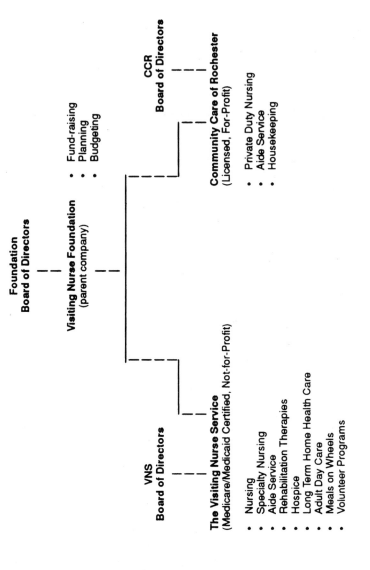

**Foundation
Board of Directors**

Visiting Nurse Foundation
(parent company)

- Fund-raising
- Planning
- Budgeting

**VNS
Board of Directors**

The Visiting Nurse Service
(Medicare/Medicaid Certified, Not-for-Profit)

- Nursing
- Specialty Nursing
- Aide Service
- Rehabilitation Therapies
- Hospice
- Long Term Home Health Care
- Adult Day Care
- Meals on Wheels
- Volunteer Programs

**CCR
Board of Directors**

Community Care of Rochester
(Licensed, For-Profit)

- Private Duty Nursing
- Aide Service
- Housekeeping

which serves as the parent company for the two subsidiary corporations, The Visiting Nurse Service and Community Care of Rochester. One of the subsidiaries is not for profit; the other is a for-profit entity. Each corporation has its own Board of Directors, with minimal overlap, and separate management teams. The scope of services includes all Medicare certified home health, both long and short term home care aide and housekeeping, continuous private duty care, hospice, home-delivered meals and adult day care. Each operating corporation hires its employees based on the services provided out of that entity; staff are not used interchangeably across corporations. The Visiting Nurse Service alone employs over 1,100 staff, while Community Care employs 200.

2. A Managed Care Organization

Group Health Cooperative of Puget Sound in Washington state is a large nonprofit staff and network model health maintenance organization, serving members spread out over six counties. Its home care services include six main program areas: home health services, hospice services, community parent/child services, home infusion therapy services, home and community volunteer services, and HIV/AIDS care coordination services. In addition, a sixth program, external delivery system, arranges and monitors home care services purchased from non Group Health providers. As indicated in Chart II, these home care services are integrated organizationally with Group Health's care management and long term care institutional services, under the same executive leadership. In this model, the administrative core functions of finance and planning, quality and care management, and information services are shared among home care, long term care and other community services.

The home care services are provided by interdisciplinary practice teams, composed of nurses, both registered and practical, rehabilitation therapists, social workers, home health aides and volunteers. These teams work out of three regional offices, with each office under the direction of an associate administrator. Certain services, such as home infusion and evening and night staffing are centralized.

CHART II. Group Health Cooperative of Puget Sound Community Health and Long Term Care

```
                                                                  ┌─────────────────────┐
                                                                  │ COMMUNITY HEALTH AND│
                                                                  │ LONG TERM CARE MEDICAL│
                                                                  │   STAFF LEADERSHIP  │
                                                                  └─────────────────────┘

          ┌──────────────┐
          │  Membership  │
          └──────────────┘
                 │
          ┌──────────────┐
          │Board of Trustees│
          └──────────────┘
                 │
          ┌──────────────┐
          │Service/Quality│
          │  Committee   │
          └──────────────┘
                 │
          ┌──────────────────┐
          │ Community Health │
          │ and Long Term Care│
          │     Council      │
          └──────────────────┘
                 │
      ┌──────────┐
      │   CEO    │
      └──────────┘
           │
      ┌──────────┐                    ┌───────────────────┐
      │VP and COO│                    │ Executive Director,│
      └──────────┘                    │ COMMUNITY HEALTH AND│
     │    │    │                      │ LONG TERM CARE (CH/LTC)│
┌──────┐┌──────┐┌──────┐              └───────────────────┘
│Regional││VP for││Assistant│
│ VPs  ││Nursing││  VPs  │
└──────┘└──────┘└──────┘

┌──────────┐┌──────────┐┌──────────────────┐┌──────────────┐┌──────────────┐┌──────────────┐
│Director, ││Director, ││ Deputy Director,  ││Manager, Quality││ Planning and ││Administrator,│
│FINANCE & ││ CH/LTC   ││ CH/LTC,          ││ Management    ││Development,  ││The Care Center│
│PLANNING  ││Care Mgmt ││ Administrator,    ││ Services      ││CH/LTC Info   ││at Kelsey Creek│
│          ││          ││ HOME CARE SERVICES,││              ││ Systems      ││              │
│          ││          ││ and Nursing       ││              ││              ││              │
│          ││          ││ Administrator,    ││              ││              ││              │
│          ││          ││ CH/LTC           ││              ││              ││              │
└──────────┘└──────────┘└──────────────────┘└──────────────┘└──────────────┘└──────────────┘
```

57

3. A Home Care Aide Organization

Cooperative Home Care Associates (CHCA), located in the South Bronx, is a for-profit, worker-owned company that provides home health aide and homemaker services. Its owner-workers are primarily African American and Latino women who live and work in Harlem and the South Bronx and who relied on public assistance prior to employment with CHCA. The workers are eligible to become owners after three months of satisfactory employment. Each share costs $1,000, which can be paid out of wages over a multiyear period. All worker-owners select the Board of Directors, who hire and fire the president. CHCA is unique as a cooperative model, designed to provide paraprofessional workers with a true sense of belonging and investment in the organization (Surpin, 1994).

CHCA's organizational structure (Chart III) reflects a streamlined, focused emphasis on their core business and highlights the importance of training and education.

INTEGRATED DELIVERY SYSTEMS FOR THE ELDERLY

We are bombarded daily with messages about the future of health care delivery: integrated services, provider networks, managed care, to name just a few. Mergers, acquisitions, joint ventures and network development strategies, while still relatively new fare within the traditional "aging network," are well-established in the home care vocabulary. This trend is fueled by the economic conditions of the health and human service fields and driven by third-party payors seeking lower costs and one-stop shopping. An equally compelling reason behind this trend, however, are the difficulties and confusion that consumers experience, particularly the older consumer with complex service needs, as they try to navigate a complicated, fragmented system. Nowhere are the difficulties more evident than in the lack of integration between acute care and long term care services for those with chronic illness and disability. Persons with chronic conditions represent the fastest growing, most complex and costly segment of the health care system; yet the way services are organized, delivered and financed continues to reflect an episodic, acute care, cure-oriented approach.

CHART III. Cooperative Home Care Associates

Table of Organization

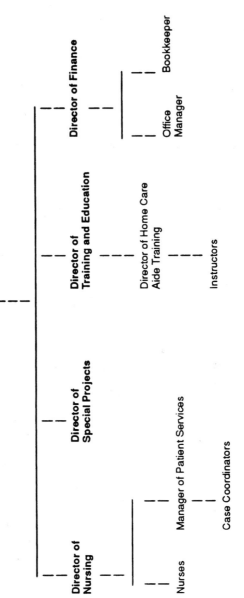

President

Director of Special Projects

Director of Training and Education

Director of Finance

Director of Nursing

Manager of Patient Services

Case Coordinators

Nurses

Director of Home Care Aide Training

Instructors

Office Manager

Bookkeeper

Cooperative Home Care Associates
New York, New York

To a great extent, home care reflects this separation between acute and long term care. The Medicare providers, focusing primarily on acute skilled home care services and the Older Americans Act and Title XX providers, delivering paraprofessional long term home care services, seem worlds apart in their organizational structures, policy perspectives, delivery mechanisms and financing.

Described below are models of integrated care delivery for the elderly and chronically impaired that are attempting to create more comprehensive, coordinated and efficient systems.

National Chronic Care Consortium (NCCC)

The NCCC is an organization of twenty-two leading health care networks dedicated to transforming the delivery of chronic care services. The NCCC believes that persons with chronic illness require an integrated continuum of primary prevention, acute, transitional, and long term care services. Its work is centered around developing local chronic care networks, which are defined as "a person-centered, systems-oriented alliance between acute and long term care providers who serve people at risk for long term disability resulting from one or more serious and persistent chronic conditions. The relationships between the system components are integrated to maintain a seamless continuum of care" (NCCC, 1994). Each network member of NCCC includes a full continuum of care, with home care services occupying a pivotal position. In these examples of vertically integrated networks, home care providers are closely linked with primary care providers, acute and long term care institutional providers in ways that encourage them to share information, utilize the same care management approaches, and develop ways to ultimately integrate financing across all levels and sites of care. The NCCC membership list is included in Chart IV.

Program of All Inclusive Care for the Elderly (PACE)

PACE is the national replication of the On Lok Senior Health Services Model developed in San Francisco and conducted by select provider sites across the country. The PACE model offers and manages the full spectrum of health, medical and social services

CHART IV

NCCC Membership ─────────────────────────────────────

Each NCCC member is a leading-edge health care provider or strategically-aligned group of providers that holds a national reputation for leadership in health care delivery and reform. NCCC members provide exemplary leadership in health care reform, sharing a commitment to excellence and the NCCC vision of integrated chronic care. NCCC members have been directly involved in virtually every major national demonstration in long-term care over the last 10 years, including On Lok replications, Social HMOs, and the Channeling Project. Each NCCC site has a complete continuum of hospital, nursing home, physician, and community-based long-term care programs.

The following organizations are NCCC members:

Amherst H. Wilder Foundation/HealthEast and UCare Minnesota, St. Paul, MN
Baylor University Medical Center, Dallas, TX
Beth Abraham Hospital, Bronx, NY
Beverly Hospital, Beverly, MA
Carondelet Health Care, Tucson, AZ
The Eddy, Troy, NY
Fairview Hospital & Healthcare Services and The Ebenezer Society, Minneapolis, MN
Fairhill (Benjamin Rose Institute and University Hospitals Health System), Cleveland, OH
Group Health Cooperative of Puget Sound, Seattle, WA
Henry Ford Health System, Detroit, MI
Huntington Memorial Hospital and Visiting Nurse Association of L.A., Pasadena/Los Angeles, CA
Intermountain Health Care, Salt Lake City, UT
Johns Hopkins Health System, Baltimore, MD
Lutheran General HealthSystem, Arlington Heights & Park Ridge, IL
Lutheran Health Systems (Lutheran Healthcare Network), Mesa, AZ
Mount Zion Institute on Aging and the University of California, San Francisco, CA
Philadelphia Geriatric Center and Albert Einstein Healthcare Network, Philadelphia, PA
Provenant Health Partners, Denver, CO
Rochester Health Care and Park Ridge Health Systems, Rochester, NY
St. Mary Medical Center, Long Beach, CA
Sentara Health System, Norfolk and Virginia Beach area, VA
Sutter Health, Sacramento, CA

The National Chronic Care Consortium • 5001 West 80th Street, Suite 449 • Bloomington, MN 55437 • (612) 835-1915 required to keep a frail elderly person as independent as possible in the community. All care is provided by one nonprofit health care organization, utilizing a community day health center as the focus for as many of the services as possible. The PACE provider receives a monthly capitation for each participant and is responsible for providing all needed health care services, including acute and long term institutional care if needed.

The organizational key to the PACE model is the multidisciplinary team, composed of the day health center staff, home care staff, and physician who make all admission and resource allocation decisions. The team bases its care decisions on participant need and the philosophy of maintaining independence and function, and does not use participant specific financial data in reaching its decisions. The day health center focus means that much of what would be provided in other settings, such as skilled nursing in the home, can be done in the center. When home care is required by enrollees in the PACE program, the majority of the service is provided by home health aides (Levesque, 1993).

LIVING AT HOME/BLOCK NURSE PROGRAM

The Living at Home/Block Nurse Program (LAH/BNP) is a Minnesota-based project designed in 1981 to develop an integrated neighborhood-based senior care model to serve elderly in their homes. The program utilizes professionals and volunteers, who are local residents, to provide information, support, social, nursing and other services to elderly persons on a neighborhood basis. Drawing heavily upon family support, neighborhood volunteers and community resources, such as churches, LAH/BNP integrates these informal services with the formal health and social service systems. It tries to build a spirit of community self-help, with both paid staff and volunteers residing in the neighborhood they serve. In so doing, LAH/BNP maintains that they can respond to needs much earlier than the traditional health care system can, offering a scope of service beyond the conventional services, at a cost less than the traditional system.

The LAH/BNP is a partnership between a home health nursing organization and a neighborhood or public entity, governed by residents from the neighborhood. The program structure consists of a program director, supervising nurse, and director of volunteers. Services for each client are arranged and coordinated by a primary block nurse or services coordinator, and delivered by a team of home health block nurses, block companions and block volunteers. By combining the functions of home health aides and homemakers into one position, the block companion, the LAH/BNP is able to offer a wider variety of services without the disruption, cost and fragmentation of conventional paraprofessional services.

The LAH/BNP identifies nine qualitative dimensions that they believe distinguish it from traditional home health care programs: client centered programming, coordination and integration of services, community-based staffing, prevention/recovery focus, early intervention, management of chronic illness/disability, delayed or reduced institutionalization, case mix openness, and fee flexibility. Data from a 1991 replication evaluation indicated that the average cost per client per month was less than $500 compared with $2000 per month nursing home costs, and 38% of the clients would be in a nursing home without the program (Jamieson, 1993).

In an era of scarce resources and expanding need, LAH/BNP holds itself out as a model of the potential for neighborhoods and communities to address the challenge of community-based long term care. The state of Minnesota is now providing some funding to assist other communities across the state to develop similar models. The Minnesota experience has led to its participation in the Community Nursing Organization Project, described below.

COMMUNITY NURSING ORGANIZATION

The Community Nursing Organization (CNO) Project is a demonstration conducted by the Health Care Financing Administration in four sites across the country. Its purpose is to design and implement a nurse-managed health care delivery system designed to improve the level of health and appropriate use of health-related services in a defined community of Medicare enrollees (CNO Consortium, 1993). Each CNO provides traditional Medicare Part A home health services, plus Medicare Part B nonphysician services such as durable medical equipment and prosthetics, outpatient physical therapy, clinical psychologist or social work counseling services and ambulance. The CNO also covers nursing case management, utilizing strategies that emphasize prevention, continuity and active consumer involvement. The CNO is paid a monthly capitation amount per Medicare enrollee, and is at risk for providing all covered services within that amount. The CNO sites are the LAH/BNP program in St. Paul, Visiting Nurse Service of New York, Carondelet Health Services, Inc., Arizona, and the Carle Clinic Association of Urbana, Illinois.

CONCLUSION

Organizational models in home care will continue to evolve as the field changes and expands. It is important to remember that there is no ideal model, since organizational form is determined by multiple factors. It is likely, however, that traditional models will be altered by integrated service delivery systems of the future, in which home care has closer organizational alignment with other levels of care in a continuum. Emerging workplace practices, such as the reduction of middle managers and the growth of self-directed work teams could significantly alter current supervisory structures. Adding to these forces are the information technology advances that expand the mechanisms by which people can work together and communicate within organizations. Taken together, these factors may result in a future organizational landscape that appears quite different. In the meantime, given the complexity and dynamism of home care, an organization's flexibility and responsiveness to change may well be the critical determinant of success.

AUTHOR NOTE

The author expresses appreciation to Jeanee Parker-Martin, RN, MPH, for her advice and review of this manuscript.

REFERENCES

California Administrative Code (1982). Licensing and certification of home health agencies. North Highlands, CA: State of California.
Community Nursing Organization Consortium (1993). "Community nursing organizations national demonstration." St. Paul, MN: Community Nursing Organization Consortium. Unpublished.

Estes, C. (1988). "Running as fast as they can: Organizational changes in home health care." In Lyman, R. and Hodgkinson, V. (Eds.). *The nonprofit sector.* San Francisco, CA: Jossey-Bass.

Home Health Assembly of New Jersey (1993). *Vision paper for home health care.* Princeton, NJ: Home Health Assembly of New Jersey.

Hughes, S. (1992). "Home care: Where we are and where we need to go." In Ory, M. and Duncker, A. (Eds.). *Home care for older people.* Newbury Park, CA: Sage Publications.

Jamieson, M. (1993). "Description of the living at home/block nurse program." St. Paul, MN: Living at Home/Block Nurse Program. Unpublished.

Levesque, R. (1993). "The PACE model: Success in cooperation," *Caring,* 10, 62-66.

National Association for Home Care (1994). *Basic statistics about home care 1994.* Washington, DC: National Association for Home Care.

National Association for Home Care (1992). *List of 101 non-traditional home care and hospice services.* Washington, DC: National Association for Home Care.

National Chronic Care Consortium (1994). *Fact sheet.* Minneapolis, MN: National Chronic Care Consortium.

Surpin, R. (1994). "Cooperative Home Care Associates." In Handy, J. and Schuerman, C. (Eds.). *Challenges and innovations in homecare.* San Francisco, CA: American Society on Aging.

Tweed, S. (1993). "Strategic focus: A game plan for collaboration in a competitive market place," *Caring,* 10, 8-14.

Yessne, P. (1994). "Home health today (part I)," *Home Health Business Report,* 1, 13-14.

Chapter 4

The Importation
of High Technology Services
into the Home

Lenard W. Kaye, DSW
Joan K. Davitt, MSS, MLSP

INTRODUCTION

This chapter presents programming strategies for agencies which are currently providing or considering the delivery of technology-enhanced home health care services (hereafter also referred to as high-tech services). Such issues as admissions criteria, staff training and supervision, administration and management, quality assurance, and patient assessment and training will be reviewed with special emphasis on elderly and disabled high-tech patients and their particular needs. The challenges, drawbacks, and benefits of high-tech services will be discussed. The final section of the chapter provides a review of some of the more "popular" high-tech services offered with a special focus on the latest innovations in in-home technology and service delivery.

In this review, high-tech home health care services will be considered to be those methods of diagnosis, treatment or rehabilitation which are embodied in or supported by specialized equipment.

[Haworth co-indexing entry note]: "The Importation of High Technology Services into the Home." Kaye, Lenard W., and Joan K. Davitt. Co-published simultaneously in *Journal of Gerontological Social Work* (The Haworth Press, Inc.) Vol. 24, No. 3/4, 1995, pp. 67-94; and: *New Developments in Home Care Services for the Elderly: Innovations in Policy, Program, and Practice* (ed: Lenard W. Kaye) The Haworth Press, Inc., 1995, pp. 67-94. Single or multiple copies of this article are available from The Haworth Document Delivery Service [1-800-342-9678, 9:00 a.m. - 5:00 p.m. (EST)].

© 1995 by The Haworth Press, Inc. All rights reserved. *67*

When defining high-tech services, it is also important to remember that home health care agency providers' views of high-tech care often reflect additional, more subtle perspectives on the properties of this special category of in-home service (Kaye and Davitt, 1994). Although many home care staff feel that the presence of specialized equipment in the home can make a service high-tech, many also feel that other factors can play an influential role in making a service high-tech. Agency providers of home health care place, in particular, special emphasis on the complexity or intensity of the treatment and the novelty of the service or treatment in identifying a particular in-home intervention as technology-enhanced. For example, a service will often be viewed as high-tech because it requires new or specialized skills on the part of the nurse or therapist. Such services as home infusion therapy, respiratory support, dialysis, artificial nutrition and hydration, and cardiac monitoring can be considered high-tech from this perspective. Additionally, novel home adaptations, such as personal emergency response systems, telecommunications systems, robotics, self-instruction computers and other "smart house" designs are seen as representing an additional layer of high-tech systems available to support a person in his/her home.

THE HIGH-TECH HOME HEALTH CARE BOOM

The rapid advance in medical treatment, including the development of new technology that allows certain types of services and equipment to be used in the home, has supported the high-tech home health care boom. Technology has been made increasingly more portable and accessible to consumers residing in their homes. At the same time, the Prospective Payment System (PPS) has aided in expanding the market for home health services generally, and high-tech in-home care in particular (Estes et al., 1993; Kaye, 1988; Kenney, 1991). Generally, patients are now being discharged from hospitals sooner and with more complex follow-up care needs than ever before. According to Estes et al. (1993), most agencies in 1986/87 were adding highly medical services to their programs, while prior to the Medicare PPS, mainly for-profit agencies were adding highly medical services. Also, Medicare-certified agencies were more likely to add highly medical services than noncertified agencies (Binney, 1990). This points to the connection between diagnosis-related groups (DRGs) and high-tech home health care. Recent research has demonstrated that home health care agency directors most frequently point to technological advances and DRGs to explain the increase in patient requests for high-tech services (Kaye and Davitt, 1994). These two factors have led to significant increases in the provision of high-tech care in the patient's home in the last seven years.

Furthermore, home health care agencies are continuing to expand the amount and variety of high-tech services offered. And, many agencies which may not currently be providing high-tech services plan to develop those services in the near future (Kaye and Davitt, 1994). This expansion is clearly driven by health care economics, and related changes in market demographics.

THE ADMINISTRATIVE CHALLENGE IN HIGH-TECH CARE

Becoming a high-tech home health care provider (or even expanding existing high-tech services) is no simple matter. There are a variety of issues which must be carefully explored prior to providing a new service or serving a new population. This is true for both traditional and high-tech services. In most cases, agencies decide to provide new services because they perceive a need or demand in their service community. For example, an agency may receive multiple requests for in-home infusion services. Of course, perceiving that a need exists is merely the first step in a complex process to define the intensity of that need in precise and accurate terms.

Conducting a needs assessment is an essential tool in the agency's development of new or expansion of existing programs. This assessment should examine the following areas:

1. agency mission;
2. target population;
3. actual need/demand for service;
4. agency internal resources to meet that demand;
5. available external resources;
6. competition from other agencies in the community; and

7. cost/benefit to deliver the service (to the agency, the community, and the client group).

The objectives of such an assessment when conducted in a given community would be to avoid the duplication of service, prevent fragmentation of the service delivery network, design an effective delivery strategy to meet the specific needs of the population, and promote long-term stability for the agency in providing the service.

The agency's mission may dictate very clearly the types of high-tech, in-home treatments that the agency can provide. For example, a hospice organization will be limited in the types of high-tech services offered due to their mission to provide palliative care. On the other hand, a proprietary home care agency may have a much more broad mission such as to serve the comprehensive health care needs of the community and would therefore be able to consider offering a wider range of high-tech interventions. It is important to be cognizant of an agency's mission and goal statement during the planning phase. Such statements might describe a specific consumer population to be targeted limiting, therefore, the types of patients an agency might serve and the range of technology-enhanced services that would be needed.

As with any legitimate service planning exercise, the identification of specific patient needs and the degree of such need within the community should occur prior to delivering the service. This is essential in order to determine accurately the amount and type of staff needed, the skills and experience required, and the degree and intensity of each service to be offered.

The needs assessment process will also shed light on the various target populations that may exist in the community and specific needs related to each target group. The needs assessment can incorporate various strategies to analyze market parameters. Such methods include community-wide surveys, key informant interviews, and monitoring actual requests for service. Much can also be learned by staying abreast of current health care trends. For example, the development of several subacute facilities in a given community may indicate the need and market for high-tech home care.

Once the need and the market have been determined, the agency must look internally to decide whether the resources exist currently to respond to the demand. Agency directors report that high-tech services have required an expansion in both the number of staff and the skill levels of staff (Kaye and Davitt, 1994). Required internal agency resources include adequate staff numbers to respond to the volume of requests, requisite staff skill levels to respond to specific service requests, fiscal stability (e.g., positive cash flow), and capacity for program evaluation and quality assurance measures to monitor actual program effectiveness and respond to market fluctuations.

Assessment of market competition serves a dual purpose. First, one can determine what services are already being provided in the community. Second, one can determine how much of the market is already being served. Agencies will want to ensure that there is enough demand for a particular service prior to offering such service directly. There are substantial costs to the agency in terms of administrative overhead, staff training, and recruitment/marketing when developing and offering new services. If demand is low, an agency may be unable to maintain fiscal stability and recoup the initial investment. Market saturation may therefore preclude an agency from offering a particular high-tech service.

Agencies may choose to be generalist in their approach to service provision or specialize in a particular service (e.g., IV antibiotics) or set of services (e.g., infusion therapies). According to Schmid and Hasenfeld (1993) a generalist strategy enables the organization to provide a more comprehensive system of care, to reach a broader target population, and to be responsive to changes in the demand for and supply of services. However, this approach is more costly, increases administrative demands, may be less efficient, and requires additional quality control. A specialist strategy, on the other hand, enables the agency to target a special population or service. Specialization reduces administrative demands (quality control issues become less burdensome) within the agency and increases efficiency. However, specialization can lead to fragmentation of the service network, thereby reducing consumer access to services and increasing service coordination costs (Schmid and Hasenfeld, 1993). Also, specialist agencies can be slow to respond to market changes. Likewise, specialization can require "complex referral, subcontracting, and special vendor relations between agencies" (Collopy et al., 1990).

Heavy competition in a specific marketplace may promote duplication, especially if most agencies choose to provide the "high-demand" service. This may be avoided by developing subcontracts with agencies that specialize in a particular service. The decision to subcontract may also be driven by a variety of other factors such as limited agency size, limited staff expertise, limited demand for service, and lack of 24-hour coverage. Subcontract arrangements do not free an agency from legal liability. An agency can in some cases be liable for actions taken by the subcontractor (see, for example, *Roach v. Kelly Health Care* 742 P2d 1190 (1987)). Monitoring procedures and quality assurance measures must be established to ensure that services are delivered effectively and efficiently.

Providing the service directly may require recruitment and hiring of new staff and/or retraining existing staff (both those who will serve direct and ancillary functions in delivering the new service). New staff may include professional groups which agency administrators have not worked with before. For example, agencies providing ventilator care may need to hire respiratory therapists to support this new treatment. This will also require updating administrative staff knowledge in a particular area in order for proper supervision to be maintained and quality assurance measures performed.

Agencies that have never offered high-tech services may want to phase-in services gradually, limiting themselves to one or two services to begin with. Marketplace competition may define more readily the boundaries in service delivery. No or very limited competition will enable an agency to take on new services more quickly. Greater competition may make it difficult to provide a full range of services at once.

Establishing Admissions Criteria

Regardless of the types of service an agency provides, admissions criteria are essential to the appropriate delivery of service to patients and to the success of any high-tech program. The pivotal aspect to all admissions, however, is conducting a complete patient assessment (Kaye and Davitt, 1994). Patient assessment consists of a determination of: (1) the staff's ability to handle patients' care needs; (2) the capacity for self-care or the availability and capability of one or more caregivers; (3) the suitability of the home environment; and (4) adequate reimbursement sources to pay for services (Larkins and Hellige, 1992).

First of all, the agency must have the resources and expertise to respond to the specific patient's care needs. The agency would need to determine whether this service had ever been offered in the past by themselves or any agency. If the service is very new or experimental for the home care arena, it would be especially important to determine whether third-party reimbursement would be available for such a service. Likewise, if the agency had never offered a particular service before, the agency would need to determine that they have the internal resources to serve such a patient (e.g., staff skills and expertise, adequate numbers of staff, 24-hour coverage). Also, it may be helpful with new or highly complex treatment modalities to provide several treatments prior to discharge from the hospital. This will help to stabilize the patient and the treatment regime before discharge, decreasing the risk of complications after discharge. Such a strategy also allows for additional time for patient/caregiver teaching.

Patients also need to be assessed to determine their (or their caregiver's) capacity for self-care. In many home care cases patients are required to monitor care and equipment, know the signs of trouble, coordinate service provision, and in many high-tech cases actually administer their own treatment (Kaye and Davitt, 1994). For example, a patient with a feeding tube may need to change the feeding at night when a nurse is not available. That same patient may be asked to monitor the insertion site for redness, swelling, or other signs of infection or to check the feeding pump to ensure that it is operating properly. Likewise, the patient needs to know how to contact the agency in case of an emergency. The availability of a caregiver and/or a highly capable and motivated patient are essential to the success of high-tech home care.

The home environment must be suitable for high-tech care. Many homes lack the necessary utilities (heat, refrigeration, running water, electricity) or storage space for high-tech care. For example, certain medications must be refrigerated or clean water may be needed to flush a feeding tube. The patient's home may be fraught with safety risks and other hazards such as unsanitary conditions, infestation, and faulty wiring. The location of the home may also make it difficult to deliver many types of services. For example, rural agencies often find themselves with patients whose homes are isolated far from the agency with limited access by automobile (Kaye and Davitt, 1994). In urban settings patient location may make it dangerous for staff as well as for the patient who may be extremely vulnerable to crime or exploitation.

Obviously, the patient must agree to home care as the preferred choice for care delivery. Most patients prefer to return to the home to recuperate from an illness. However, there may be a patient on occasion who will request placement in a long-term care facility. Therefore, it should never be assumed that the patient will automatically choose home care. All options should be explored with the hospital patient prior to discharge.

Finally, a thorough review of the patient's financial resources and health care coverage must be conducted. Approval from the insurance provider must be obtained prior to initiating services in the home in order to protect the agency's fiscal stability. Generally, most third-party insurers, including Medicare, require a physician's prescription for home care to be covered. Without this approval the insurance company may deny coverage. Providing services without prior approval can increase the likelihood that the agency will become financially responsible and must attempt to obtain payment directly from the client. If the client is unable to pay, services may have to be terminated at a time when the client is most vulnerable, creating an ethical dilemma for agency staff.

Dealing with Reimbursement Issues

Denial of coverage has been frequently documented in the literature as one of the major barriers to quality, comprehensive home health care (Mehlman, 1991; Larkins and Hellige, 1992; Kaye, 1992; Dombi, 1992; and Collopy et al., 1992). Insurers can deny coverage altogether, deny coverage for professional services, or dispute the duration and frequency of care (Dombi, 1992). Reimbursement issues are especially important in high-tech care due to the novelty of many treatments (Kaye and Davitt, 1994). If the patient has private insurance, such as an HMO, it is appropriate for the agency to review the request for home care with the insurer in advance. At this time it would be wise to receive a written statement articulating the specific benefits offered, the duration of each benefit, and any eligibility criteria which might reduce or eliminate a particular benefit. For example, a patient may not have coverage for physical therapy to be provided in the home. They may only be covered for skilled nursing care and will need to attend outpatient physical therapy. It is essential to review the insurance package and to determine what is covered in advance, but it is most important to get it in writing.

Likewise, insurance companies may be limited by state or federal regulations related to the delivery of health care in general or home health care in particular (Dombi, 1992). Such regulations may dictate that certain services be delivered by a recognized professional. Therefore, the insurance company could not require the substitution of a paraprofessional in situations which require a professional. Agency administrators must be aware of these regulations in order to protect and advocate for patients.

As with state regulations, agency administrators must familiarize themselves with Medicare and Medicaid regulations. New treatment modalities may not be covered under Medicare and/or Medicaid, especially if they are viewed as experimental or have never been provided in the home before. Administrators will need to stay current on eligibility criteria and reimbursement procedures to ensure sound fiscal management. (For a more detailed description of home health entitlements and other benefits see Chapter 1.) High-tech services are, generally, much more costly than traditional services. Therefore, it is essential to determine in advance how much reimbursement will be available for a particular service and a particular patient. Continuing to serve high-tech patients who have exhausted insurance coverage will place a severe fiscal strain on the agency (a practice which occurs quite often with traditional home care patients). Payment sources must be a part of each patient assessment to enable the agency to continue to provide adequate services to the client in the home and maintain the patient in a safe environment.

In some cases, patients may be eligible for custodial services in conjunction with skilled services. For example, Medicare will pay for home health aide services as long as there is a need for skilled nursing services. Likewise, some states are using the Medicaid waiver program to extend in-home services and delay institutionalization by expanding the available amount of service. This, however, is not being offered in every state. It is therefore the administrator's responsibility to understand eligibility criteria to ensure that the patient receives the maximum level of service.

Program Management in the High-Tech Agency

The increased use of technology and highly skilled services in the home only emphasizes the need for expanded quality assurance strategies in each home health care agency. Every good home health care program has established procedures and protocols for staff to follow. The development of good policies promotes consistency across agency staff and ensures quality service. Important policy areas which warrant procedures and internal protocols when serving high-tech patients include: admissions criteria and client assessment; alternate coverage and emergency response procedures; termination of service; staff training and continuing education; care planning and client participation; assessment of client decision-making capacity and ability to participate in life-sustaining and other treatment decisions; and assessment of potential abuse, neglect, or exploitation.

Staffing Your High-Tech Program

In order to provide high-tech services, many agencies will need to recruit and hire new staff. This may include new professional categories (e.g., respiratory therapist) or new staff within the same profession (e.g., registered nurses) but with specialized skills. The type of staff recruited will depend on whether staff will be specialized or generalist. For example, an agency may decide to offer IV antibiotics as a new service. In order to provide this service, existing staff must be retrained or special skills staff will have to be hired. Specialization obviously promotes the most intensive knowledge and skill related to a service. However, generic staffing provides more flexibility in relation to staff coverage, emergency response, and staff turnover.

Whether or not staff specialize in certain high-tech treatment modalities will depend on the size of the agency, its service area, and the demand for high-tech services. For example, it is common for there to be a heavy demand in many communities for infusion therapies–mainly antibiotics and pain management. In this case, staff specializing in each type of infusion therapy may not be needed. On the other hand, if a particular community reflects a more varied demand for high-tech services including infusion therapy, respiratory therapy, renal dialysis, and cardiac telemetry, there would be a greater need for specialization. It would be unrealistic to expect all staff to be able to handle all of these situations.

In providing high-tech services, administrators may find themselves working with a much broader range of professional staff as well as paraprofessional staff. This may indicate additional training for administrators since they will need a more detailed understanding of service delivery. In addition, working with multiple disciplines within the same organization and on the same patient can make patient care planning ever more complicated. Administrative demands are more challenging when working with multiple disciplines. For example, staff may have very diverse training needs related to their respective disciplines. Team meetings and multi-disciplinary case reviews may help to eliminate some of the confusion and miscommunication which might occur under these circumstances. It is important for all staff to be aware of each other's differing perspectives on patient care so that interaction among staff does not become confrontational. Coordinating multiple disciplines working on the same case can demand much administrative skill and time. Kaye (1992) notes several areas which administrators should be aware of when working with multidisciplinary staff:

1. reducing the presence of potential communication barriers due to the use of discipline-specific jargon;
2. recognizing socioeconomic and cultural differences among staff;
3. extending respect to all staff for their differing skills and interests;
4. acknowledging professional "turf";
5. mediating conflicts among staff; and
6. resolving interprofessional power struggles and mediating the professional hierarchy.

It is the administrator's responsibility to ensure that the client's well-being takes precedence over any interprofessional conflicts among agency staff. These issues become even more complex when dealing with high-tech services, since generally there will be more staff involved with a high-tech patient than with the traditional home care patient.

Administrators should be aware of various other diversity issues with staff. Agency administrators will be dealing with multiple disciplines, multiple cultural backgrounds, professional vs. paraprofessional staff orientations to care, etc. Each staff person will bring a different set of life experiences into his/her work with patients. Administrators must master the skills which allow such experience to be used positively in helping the patient. Administrators also must know how to show staff when their own cultural background may be interfering with their objectivity and therefore their service to the patient. For example, during a supervisory session a staff member may express dismay at family members who have chosen to provide little assistance for a patient. The staff member is upset because he/she feels it is the responsibility of the family to care for this patient. The supervisor in this situation has the responsibility to point out to the staff person what biases may be inherent in his/her position and what underlying assumptions he/she may be making regarding this family's history and the relationship that the patient historically has had with family members.

These types of sensitive issues can be incorporated in ongoing staff training. Staff will regularly need to update their skills and their knowledge of certain treatments or services. They may also need training on working with other professionals, such as communication, case sharing, and interdisciplinary support. All staff possess unique skills which are essential to an efficient and effective service. This should be stressed throughout all orientation and staff training.

The administrator's role for ensuring quality does not end once staff have been hired. Training is essential to the best practice of high-tech services. According to Lindeman (1992), nurses need training on the use of equipment, the use of monitoring and recording devices, patient education, making clinical decisions in conditions of ambiguity, and dealing with ethical dilemmas and conflict.

Treatment modalities change rapidly in the high-tech world. Likewise, high-tech equipment is constantly changing thereby making some equipment more complex to operate. Therefore, staff skills will need to be updated on a fairly regular basis to ensure that staff are providing timely and informed assistance to patients.

More importantly, staff are responsible for teaching patients how to monitor or operate equipment and how to administer and/or monitor certain treatments. Since many patients (and/or their caregivers) are expected to monitor and even directly participate in their treatment (Kaye and Davitt, 1994), staff limitations in terms of understanding treatment procedures can be expected to impact negatively on patient understanding of those same procedures. If patients are not adequately informed regarding their treatment, side effects, and proper use of equipment, emergencies will be more likely to arise.

Training should be provided to all agency staff, not just those nurses who may be the primary deliverers of high-tech services. Social workers, homemakers/home health aides, occupational and physical therapists, case managers, and their supervisors find that they frequently serve an ancillary role in high-tech service delivery. Overall, home health aides provide more hours of service to patients than any other category of home health care staff (Kaye and Davitt, 1994). Home health aides are more likely to be in the home when an emergency occurs than any other agency staff person. They also provide much supplementary support to the high-tech patient. Home health aides provide many services including monitoring temperature, pulse, and respiration; irrigating foley catheters; and assisting with self-administered medications (Mehlman and Youngner, 1991). Therefore, they need training on emergency procedures, equipment use, and symptom recognition, as well as on any specific treatments they may be involved in providing (Liebig, 1988; Collopy et al., 1990; Kaye, 1992; Lindeman, 1992).

Agency administrators who provide high-tech services must establish a system for 24-hour coverage, as well as a back-up system to cover for staff who take leave. This is an essential prerequisite for a successful high-tech program and is one of the most difficult aspects of administering such a program according to high-tech providers (Kaye and Davitt, 1994). It is also the agency's responsibility to ensure that patients with equipment in their homes have some system for back-up power in the event of power failure. Some agencies have established regular communication with their utility companies to inform them of the location of patients with life-support equipment (e.g., ventilator, feeding tube) which operates on electricity. This way they can respond to that patient more quickly or, if the power outage is to be extended, they can make arrangements to admit the patient to a health care institution as quickly as possible.

Agency administrators are more and more frequently finding themselves in the dilemma of balancing client need against employee safety. Both the location and the condition of a patient's home may place agency staff at risk. The home health care agency owes a duty to employees to protect them from injury as they carry out their responsibilities on the agency's behalf. A variety of factors can place staff at risk in the high-tech arena. These include work with toxic substances (e.g., chemotherapy agents), working with body fluids, exposure to contagious agents (e.g., tuberculosis, hepatitis), travel during inclement weather or at night, and unsafe neighborhoods or patient homes. Injury may include contracting a contagious disease or being injured en route to a patient's home, in operation of equipment, or otherwise within the patient's home. Likewise, under the Freedom of Information Act and federal labor laws, staff have a right to know if any materials that they work with may be hazardous. Staff who provide IV chemotherapy in the home can be exposed to health risks and must be properly trained in the handling of hazardous chemicals. Appropriate policies should be established to ensure that decisions regarding employee safety are made consistently, and afford the opportunity for direct administrative review (e.g., supervisor going to site with staff).

Universal precautions must be stressed with staff in teaching patients and caregivers (including proper disposal of biohazards or toxic materials). In addition, appropriate infection control procedures must be taught to patients and their caregivers. As mentioned earlier, if staff are not using proper aseptic procedures and universal precautions it is likely that patients and their caregivers will not use them as well. How-to clinical references for high-tech home care therapies are now available to support an agency's efforts in this area (Gorski, 1994).

High-Tech Client Assessment and Education

Home care staff are providing service to individuals who are older, more debilitated, and increasingly dependent on others for life maintenance (Kaye and Davitt, 1994). This trend in home care consumer demographics only magnifies the need for thorough client assessment. Assessment includes a complete evaluation of the patient including cognitive status, functional ability, motivation/ emotional well-being, ability to learn, financial status (including the availability of third-party coverage), and informal support.

As with all medical procedures, patients are entitled to provide informed consent. Therefore, prior to initiating service, home care patients should be informed about the purpose of the treatment, the benefits and drawbacks to treatment, treatment alternatives, specific risks related to home treatment, limitations of service, self-care requirements, and patient financial liability. At a minimum, patient education should include knowledge of the disease process; understanding of self-care tasks and regimen; explanation of proper procedures during emergencies (including appropriate emergency contact numbers, equipment use, and preventive activities); and recognizing signs and symptoms of problems (Grieco, 1991; Smith, 1992; Liebig, 1988; Worcester, 1990). Patient education is important to preventing agency liability. The need for documentation of patient/ caregiver education is just as important as direct care documentation (McAbee, 1991).

The provision of high-tech equipment and services in the home can pose a number of ethical and legal challenges for both the older patient and the agency. Because the use of high-tech procedures are making it possible for people with chronically acute conditions to live longer, it is not unusual for questions surrounding patient's rights, right to die, delegation of authority, competency, death, and dying to arise during the course of home care service delivery (Arras, 1995; Kaye and Davitt, 1994). Agency participation in patient and family decisions related to foregoing life-sustaining treatment, preparing living wills, and using durable powers of attorney and guardians is not uncommon.

Patient education around a person's right to execute advance directives is now required under the federal Patient Self-Determination Act. Agencies can encourage patient participation in their own plan of care by explaining their rights as patients upon entry into the program, involving them in plan-of-care conferences, actively seeking feedback from patients and their families, and providing information to patients about their care on a regular basis. By educating patients on the benefits of advance directives, agencies can reduce the number of later conflicts over life-sustaining treatment decisions if a patient becomes incapacitated.

Home health care agencies are also encouraged to consider establishing, if they have not already done so, policies regarding how staff should handle decisions about life-sustaining treatment as well as policies for dealing with patients who have questionable decision-making capacity. Home care agencies can avail themselves of a variety of programs and policies for dealing with the legal and ethical demands of delivering high-tech care including in-service training for staff; encouraging staff to attend community continuing education and training programs; organizing plan-of-care conferences with staff, families, and patients; organizing special staff meetings and supervisory sessions geared to particular thematic issues; and developing customized information systems for documenting high-tech service delivery. Other strategies for agencies to consider include the use of ethics committees and ethicists, legal counsel and consultants, and educational programming for patients and their families.

Home care staff report that many patients are intimidated by equipment and that this impacts their ability to do self-care (Kaye and Davitt, 1994). Patient or caregiver fear of technology can have a direct impact on their ability to learn. Infusion services, in particular, appear to provoke much anxiety on the part of patients. When patients are anxious or otherwise preoccupied, their ability to absorb and remember important treatment details is greatly reduced. Patient teaching, therefore, must begin by reducing patient anxiety about the nature of the treatment and the safety of receiving it at home.

When teaching older patients, one must also consider any physical problems which may interfere with learning such as hearing, vision, or reading impairments. Likewise, psychosocial variables such as depression, pain, anxiety, and fatigue can interfere with learning. The patient may also have physical barriers such as mobility and dexterity problems and cognitive impairments which limit the ability to carry out self-care tasks. Such problems may require staff to develop creative strategies to teach self-care (Kaye and Davitt, 1994). Worcester (1987) suggests the following strategies when teaching older adults:

1. allow the patient to control the pace of learning;
2. begin with what the patient knows–clear up misconceptions;
3. use repetition;
4. check understanding before changing topics;
5. limit amount of material presented;
6. use large print, pictures, contrasting colors, magnifying aids;
7. use audio aids, eliminate background noise;
8. have patient demonstrate by performing task or repeating steps; and
9. provide adaptive devices to enhance patient abilities.

Different patients will have different needs, resources, and coping strategies. Therefore, agency staff must be creative in how they approach patient teaching.

INNOVATIONS IN HIGH-TECH TREATMENT

The remainder of this chapter will highlight a few of the latest innovations in high-tech medical care which can be provided at home including cardiac care, infusion therapy, artificial nutrition and hydration, and personal emergency response systems.

The most frequently provided high-tech home health care services are infusion therapies (artificial nutrition and hydration, antibiotics, pain management, and chemotherapy) (Kaye and Davitt, 1994). As previously discussed, the boundaries of high-tech care are changing continually. However, high-tech home care is generally classified in two categories: (1) medical services, treatment, and equipment, and (2) home adaptations and environmental designs.

In-Home Cardiac Services

Home care agencies may find themselves increasingly providing follow-up care for patients with cardioverter defibrillators. Many of the patients receiving such devices are over age 60. Approximately 20% of all sudden cardiac death (SCD) victims survive the initial arrest (Davidson, VanRiper, Harper, Wenk, 1994). Many survivors of SCD develop potentially fatal ventricular arrhythmias (Arato, Biggs, and Williams, 1992). The cardioverter defibrillator is used with patients who have ventricular arrhythmias (tachyarrhythmias) which are not treatable through current pharmacologic therapy. The device, pioneered by Dr. Michel Mirowski, was first used in 1980 and received FDA approval in 1985 under the name Automatic Implantable Cardioverter Defibrillator (AICD, CPI, St. Paul, Minn.).

The technical components of AICDs have improved dramatically since their creation. The two major advances include the development of multifunctional AICDs and the nonthoracotomy lead (NTL) system (Davidson et al., 1994). The nonthoracotomy lead reduces operative trauma and risk. Initial units simply detected arrhythmias and provided cardioversion/defibrillation or shocking. Current units and those still in clinical trials display significantly greater capacity including the ability to pace the patient out of tachycardia (antitachycardia pacing or ATP), cardioversion/defibrillation, and bradycardia pacing (Davidson et al., 1994).

Elderly AICD patients present a unique challenge to home care nurses and it is highly likely that their numbers will increase dramatically in the future. AICD patients have serious psychological needs after implantation such as fear of sudden death from the arrhythmia, fear of shocking, fear of "overshocking," and fear of deteriorating health and loss of independence. Lifestyle changes may also be required such as driving restrictions and avoiding environmental hazards which may affect the unit both in the workplace and the home. Patients require a great deal of nursing care both before and after implantation as well as regular follow-up care for the rest of their lives.

Discharge teaching and emotional support is essential for AICD patients and should always include significant others in the teaching sessions since the patient will generally not be able to summon help if the arrhythmia is not converted. Patient/family teaching consists of learning about the underlying disease, rhythm disturbances, the device and how it functions, postoperative care, and monitoring for signs of system malfunction and/or changes in the disease itself. In addition, patients may experience anxiety regarding the "shock sensation." Nurses can reduce this fear by discussing how other patients have described the sensation. Nurses may suggest that patients become involved in support groups or meet with other AICD patients to reduce patient anxiety post discharge.

Home care nursing staff must have knowledge of the device, the therapies to expect when an arrhythmia occurs, proper procedures for suspending therapy if the patient is shocked inappropriately, and procedures for emergency intervention should the device fail to convert the patient's rhythm (i.e., advanced cardiac life support protocols).

It is recommended that AICD patients have some type of emergency response system in place when they return home. Likewise, the hospital should provide the patient with a temporary AICD identification card and should assist the patient in applying for a Medic Alert bracelet. Patients must notify the physician every time the device fires and should keep a log including the date, time, the activity, and symptoms preceding each firing (Arato et al., 1992). Family members are encouraged to obtain instruction in CPR. Patients must avoid strong magnetic fields and high-frequency electrical sources and must learn how to recognize the effect of such fields on the device (strong magnets can deactivate the devices).

Patients must be seen in clinic or physician's office every 2-4 months depending on the device and its ability to hold a charge. Batteries last from 3-5 years but can be drained faster by frequent or excessive shocks. Changes in patient health or arrhythmia may warrant reprogramming or new medication.

This treatment is considered high-tech because of its novelty, its increasing complexity, its volatile nature, and the degree of medical knowledge and nursing training necessary to monitor patients successfully.

Points to remember:

1. Patient should have a responsible caregiver and an emergency response system in the home in the event the AICD fails to convert.
2. Patient/caregiver education is essential to reduce anxiety and ensure proper emergency response.
3. Home/work site evaluation must be conducted prior to discharge to rule out potential environmental hazards (especially magnetic fields).

Home Infusion Therapy

The most common types of infusion therapy provided by home care agencies are pain management, nutrition and hydration, antibiotics, and chemotherapy (Kaye and Davitt, 1994). Currently, there are four types of venous access devices: (1) percutaneous central catheters; (2) peripherally inserted central catheters (PICC); (3) tunnelled central venous catheters; and (4) totally implanted venous access ports. The percutaneous central catheter is most often used for short-term venous access. Insertion sites include subclavian, jugular, and femoral. The PICC is considered appropriate for infusion greater than 10-14 days and can be used for antibiotics, blood sampling, chemotherapy, fluids, palliative care, parenteral nutrition, and drugs (Ryder, 1993). The PICC line is inserted above the antecubital space and terminates in the distal superior vena cava (Ryder, 1993). The advantages to PICC lines include reduced risk of infection and air embolism, preservation of upper extremity veins, elimination of repeated venipuncture, reduced cost, and increased efficiency (Ryder, 1993). According to Ryder, the PICC line is not suited for high-fluid volume infusions, rapid bolus injection, or hemodialysis.

The external tunneled right atrial catheter is more suited for long-term access for patients who require repeated, intensive supportive therapy, infusion of vesicant chemotherapy, or long-term nutritional support (Freedman and Bosserman, 1993). The tunnelled catheter is implanted by surgical procedure under anesthesia preferably in the superior vena cava. The two main types of tunneled catheters are Hickman/Broviac and Groshong.

Totally implanted venous access ports or implanted vascular access devices (IVADs) consist of two parts, the catheter and the port.

The catheter is inserted into a large vein and is connected to the port which is implanted under the skin. The port is a self-sealing chamber which allows access to the catheter. The IVAD can be used for IV, intra-arterial, or intraperitoneal delivery of drugs and fluids (Gullo, 1993). According to Gullo the benefits to this system include allowing for a completely closed system, eliminating the need for daily site care, reducing the risk of infection, reducing the cost, and allowing for a more normal lifestyle for the patient.

Agency administrators have noted several concerns when establishing a home infusion service. They include agency ability to provide 24-hour coverage, nurse education and skill level, acceptable levels of reimbursement, and difficulty with physicians (McAbee, 1991; Kaye and Davitt, 1994). Thorough discharge planning and client admissions criteria are essential to the safe and appropriate delivery of home IV therapy. The following factors must be evaluated for each patient:

1. client/caregiver capability for self-care;
2. safe home environment;
3. stabilization of treatment prior to discharge;
4. staffing level/abilities; and
5. reimbursement issues.

Client and caregiver education is also very important since staff will not always be available in the home. In addition, the agency should have clearly established protocols and standards of practice for each type of infusion therapy.

Artificial Nutrition and Hydration Therapies

One of the most common forms of home infusion therapy is artificial nutrition and hydration, commonly known as tube feeding. There are two possible routes for delivering nutrition and water to patients who are unable to swallow, digest, or absorb food: (1) enteral nutrition and (2) parenteral nutrition. Enteral methods are used when the patient has a functioning gastrointestinal (GI) tract which is capable of absorbing nutrients and digesting food (Mehlman and Youngner, 1991; Shuster and Mancino, 1994). Enteral methods provide nutrition directly into the stomach or intestine via tubes.

Enteral tube feeding, although safer than parenteral, is not completely risk free. As with any invasive procedure there is the potential for infection especially at the insertion site. The site should be properly cleansed with proper aseptic procedures. The most important complication is the risk of vomiting and pulmonary aspiration (Aspen, 1993). This can be reduced by proper monitoring of the patient, preparation, and administration of the formula to reduce delays in gastric emptying. In addition, the patient can suffer from metabolic complications, including excess or deficient nutrients. Finally, there can be mechanical problems with the feeding tube or pump.

Patients discharged home with enteral feeding must be evaluated by a multidisciplinary team of professionals. The criteria for home tube feeding include:

1. inability to meet nutritional requirements orally;
2. clinically stable for home discharge;
3. demonstrated tolerance to the formula and schedule; and
4. patient/caregiver capacity for self-care (Aspen, 1993).

Patient monitoring must be provided by nutritional support specialists more frequently, immediately after discharge. As with all home care services, patient education is essential. Older adults have shown significantly improved understanding of this complex medical procedure following the receipt of information (Krynski, Tymchuk and Ouslander, 1994). In many cases the patient will be required to administer the feeding including mixing, changing the bag, cleaning the insertion site, and flushing the tube. The patient should be aware of aseptic procedures to prevent infection.

Parenteral feeding is used when the patient does not have a functioning GI tract or when a particular disease process interferes with absorption of food and fluids. This form of nutritional support provides nutrients and hydration through venous access. There are two types of parenteral nutrition, peripheral and central. Peripheral parenteral nutrition (PPN) is not the route of choice for individuals who require long-term nutritional support, have severe malnutrition, or have large nutrient or electrolyte needs (Worthington, 1989). Central venous access is generally used for patients who have prolonged need for nutritional support. Most patients on home parenteral nutrition (HPN) will receive nutrients through a large central vein using a catheter.

Patients must be thoroughly evaluated before HPN can be administered. Criteria for HPN are basically the same as with enteral nutrition except that the patient should be unable to meet nutritional requirements orally or unable to absorb food and fluids through the GI tract.

Again, patient teaching is essential since many HPN patients are cycled at night. The patient therefore may be responsible for changing the catheter site dressing, adding to the feeding solution, connecting the infusion to the catheter, programming the pump, redressing the entry site, disconnecting and flushing the catheter, and irrigating a blocked catheter (Friend, 1992).

Personal Emergency Response Systems

The ability to garner immediate assistance in an emergency is an important concern to anyone in our society. This concern is especially relevant to many older adults who may live alone, or be left alone for lengthy periods of time. Home care patients in particular are especially vulnerable when they return home. The electronic form of personal emergency response systems (PERS) has been available for about 10-15 years. The PERS device generally uses some type of portable radio transmitter which sends a signal to an emergency response center upon activation by the patient. The patient usually wears a tiny transmitter around his/her neck (pendant) or as a bracelet. When activated, the transmitter sends a signal through the telephone line to a central response station. This station can then perform a number of functions such as calling the patient, contacting neighbors or family, or calling local fire and rescue/ambulance services.

Manufacturers have greatly improved the capabilities and reliability of PERS over the years and such devices are now in use around the world (Tinker, 1992; Vlaskamp, 1992). For example, many companies provide a fail-safe response mechanism. If the person is unusually inactive for a certain period of time, the monitor will signal the response center (Dibner, 1990). Newer systems offer two-way voice communication. The patient is able to speak with the response center within seconds of activating the unit. Many systems also allow the patient to use the unit to answer the telephone from anywhere in the home. This is especially helpful for individuals with severe mobility impairments (e.g., quadriplegics or stroke victims). Other systems offer smoke detection and monitoring of home medical equipment.

The help buttons have also been improved. They have been made smaller, waterproof, shock resistant, and lightweight. Adaptations have been devised to make the units accessible to even the most restricted quadriplegic (Dibner, 1990).

PERS have been shown to be cost effective, promoting decreased use of the formal service system (Coordinated Care Management Corporation, 1987; Dixon, 1987).

Many patients can benefit from some form of personal emergency response. The main drawback to PERS is choosing the system that is best suited for a given patient. It is important to be aware of the variety of services which serve the geographic area of your clients. Keller (1993) provides a series of tips on choosing a PERS:

1. Investigate the system manufacturer.
2. Determine in advance how the system will be serviced and make sure there is a 24-hour response for service.
3. Test the system prior to signing a contract.
4. Determine who will monitor the signals (it should be certified professionals).
5. Make sure that central system monitors are senior-oriented, caring, and social in nature.
6. Local does not necessarily mean better.
7. Determine the level of response for each call (e.g., ambulance or family/neighbor).
8. Ask for special, state-of-the-art features such as speaker phone, smoke detectors, equipment monitors, etc.
9. Inspect the help button: is it lightweight, waterproof, simple to use?
10. Understand the philosophy of the monitoring group (i.e., do they charge for false alarms or encourage users to test the system often?).
11. Find out the cost and what is included in the cost. Higher prices do not necessarily mean better quality.

The American Association of Retired Persons has produced a product report which reviews 20 different PERS and discusses their performance (American Association of Retired Persons, 1992).

Other Technology-Enhanced Innovations

Additional categories of technology-enhanced home health care interventions, while not widely offered by agencies currently, can be expected to become more common in the years ahead as the costs associated with their use continue to drop. Included here are technologies that are not directly associated with a particular piece of medical equipment, but rather make heavy use in the home of adaptive computer hardware, software and positioning devices for older adults with chronic health problems including in-home robotics and sensory stimulation devices (O'Leary, Mann, and Perkash, 1991). Research already suggests that, contrary to stereotypical views of the elderly, most older adults are quite receptive to various computer technologies including: using personal computers generally, programming, working with applications software and recreational computer games, and communicating by means of computers (Office of Technology Assessment, 1985).

Robotics, when properly developed, have the capacity to help homebound persons in performing activities of daily living. Voice-activated personal robots are already capable of assisting impaired elders and other disabled persons with lifting, bathing, and feeding (Haber, 1986).

Home-based computer instruction technologies have application value in the areas of health promotion, improving social interaction, and even mental functioning of patients. Computer-assisted health instruction, already widely used in institutional health care settings to instruct diabetic, post-stroke, and heart disease patients, are finding their way more recently into nontraditional, community-based care settings. Computer-assisted health instruction represents a logical extension of the self-care/self-help movement in the areas of health maintenance and disease management.

At the administrative level, computer-based processing applications are being used increasingly for monitoring the health status of acutely ill or severely incapacitated older adults. At the heart of these medical monitoring innovations are interactive telecommunications systems established between the home care or other health care provider agency's office and the patient's home.

These and other technological innovations can be expected to become more widely available to the functionally impaired, community-based elderly population as the capacity and commitment to meeting the health and health-related needs of persons outside of traditional medical care settings increases. The home health care agency is positioned strategically to serve a central role in making such innovation accessible to the older adult. In so doing, home health care providers will be encouraging elders to assume greater involvement in their own health maintenance as home environments are designed to maximize an individual's functional independence.

REFERENCES

American Association of Retired Persons. (1992). "PERS (personal emergency response system)," *Product Report*, 2, 1-14.

American Society for Parenteral and Enteral Nutrition. (1993). "Guidelines for the use of parenteral and enteral nutrition in adult and pediatric patients," *Journal of Parenteral and Enteral Nutrition*, 17, 1SA-26SA.

Arato, A., Biggs, A.J., and Williams, J. (1992). "Elderly care: Automatic implantable cardioverter defibrillators," *Journal of Gerontological Nursing*, December, 15-22.

Arras, J.D. (Ed.). (1995). *Bringing the Hospital Home: Ethical and Social Implications of High-Tech Home Care*. Baltimore, MD: The Johns Hopkins University Press.

Binney, E.A., Estes, C.L., and Ingman, S.R. (1990). "Medicalization, public policy and the elderly: Social service in jeopardy?", *Social Science and Medicine*, 30, 761-771.

Collopy, B.A., Dubler, N., and Zuckerman, C. (1990). "The ethics of home care: Autonomy and accommodation," *The Hastings Center Report*, March/April, Supp., 1-16.

Coordinated Care Management Corp. (1987). *Emergency Response System Demonstration Project: Preliminary Report*. Buffalo, NY: CCMC.

Davidson, T. (1994). "Implantable cardioverter defibrillators: A guide for clinicians," *Heart and Lung*, 23, 205-215.

Dibner, A.S. (1990). "Personal emergency response systems: Communication technology aids elderly and their families," *The Journal of Applied Gerontology*, 9, 504-510.

Dixon, L. (1987). *Evaluation of Electronic Call Device Pilot Project*. New York, NY: City of New York HRA Medical Assistance Program.

Dombi, W. (1992). "Chronic intensive home care," *Caring Magazine*, March, 58-63.

Estes, C.L., Swan, J.H., and Associates. (1993). *The Long Term Care Crisis: Elders Trapped in the No-Care Zone.* Newbury Park, CA: Sage Publications, Inc.

Freedman, S. and Bosserman, G. (1993). "Tunneled catheters: Technological advances and nursing care issues," *Nursing Clinics of North America*, 851-857.

Friend, B. (1992). "Self-service," *Nursing Times*, 88, 26-28.

Gorski, L.A. (1994). *High-Tech Home Care Manual.* Frederick, MD: Aspen Publishers.

Grieco, A.J. (1991). "Physician's guide to managing home care of older patients," *Geriatrics*, 46, 49-60.

Gullo, S. (1993). "Implanted ports: Technological advances and nursing care issues," *Nursing Clinics of North America*, 28, 859-870.

Haber, P.A.L. (1986). "Technology in aging," *The Gerontologist*, 26, 350-357.

Kaye, L.W. (1988). "Generational equity: Pitting young against old," *New England Journal of Human Services*, 8, 8-11.

Kaye, L.W. (1992). *Home Health Care.* Newbury Park, CA: Sage Publications.

Kaye, L.W. and Davitt, J.K. (1994). *High-Tech Home Health Care: An Analysis of Service Delivery and Consumption, Final Report to the AARP Andrus Foundation.* Bryn Mawr, PA: Bryn Mawr College.

Keller, S.R. (1993). "A guide to personal emergency response systems," *Answers*, 2, 12-32.

Kenney, G.M. (1991). "Understanding the effects of PPS on Medicare home health use," *Inquiry*, 28, 129-139.

Krynski, M.D., Tymchuk, A.J. and Ouslander, J.G. (1994). "How informed can consent be? New light on comprehension among elderly people making decisions about enteral tube feeding," *The Gerontologist*, 34, 36-43.

Larkins, F.R., and Hellige, M. (1992). "Adding high-tech home care services to your agency," *Caring Magazine*, September, 18-22.

Liebig, P.S. (1988). "The use of high technology for health care at home: Issues and implications," *Medical Instrumentation*, 22, 222-225.

Lindeman, C.A. (1992). "Nursing and technology: Moving into the 21st century," *Caring Magazine*, September, 5-17.

McAbee, R.R., Grupp, K., and Horn, B. (1991). "Home intravenous therapy: Part I–Issues," *Home Health Care Services Quarterly*, 12, 59-108.

Mehlman, M.J., and Youngner, S.J. (1991). *Delivering High Technology Home Care.* New York, NY: Springer Publishing Company.

Office of Technology Assessment, Congress of the United States. (1985). *Technology and Aging in America.* Washington, DC: U.S. Government Printing Office.

O'Leary, S., Mann, C. and Perkash, I. (1991). "Access to computers for older adults: Problems and solutions," *American Journal of Occupational Therapy*, 45, 636-642.

Ryder, M. (1993). "Peripherally inserted central venous catheters," *Nursing Clinics of North America*, 28, 937-971.

Schmid, H. and Hasenfeld, Y. (1993). "Organizational dilemmas in the provision of home care services," *Social Service Review*, March, 41-53.

Shuster, M.H. and Mancino, J.M. (1994). "Ensuring successful home tube feeding in the geriatric population," *Geriatric Nursing*, 15, 67-81.

Smith, S. (1992). "Advanced states," *Nursing Times*, 88, 31-32.

Tinker, A. (1992). "Alarms and telephones in emergency response–Research from the United Kingdom," *Home Health Care Services Quarterly*, 13, 177-189.

Vlaskamp, F.J. (1992). "From alarm systems to smart houses," *Home Health Care Services Quarterly*, 13, 105-122.

Worcester, M.I. (1990). "Tailoring teaching to the elderly in home care." In *Facilitating Self Care Practices in the Elderly*. New York, NY: The Haworth Press, Inc.

Worcester, M.I. (1987). *Tailoring Teaching to the Elderly in the Home*. University of Washington Institute on Aging.

Worthington, P.H. (1989). "Total parenteral nutrition," *Nursing Clinics of North America*, 24, 355-371.

Chapter 5

Home Health Care Information Systems: Difficult Choices in Uncertain Times

Dick Schoech, PhD
Janet Neff, RN, BSN
Karen Roberts, MSSW

INTRODUCTION

An old saying exists that you can tell the pioneers by the arrows in their backs. This saying aptly describes the dangers in home care information system (IS) development. Yet, a good, up-to-date IS is essential for home care agency survival. Home care providers must make IS choices, yet the home care system is changing and will continue to change given today's emphasis on managed care and reform. In addition, home care ISs are not developed to the extent of other ISs in the health delivery system. This is because the home care field has been in existence only a short time and a standard home care delivery system does not exist. Consequently, home care providers in charge of IS development are true pioneers who must make risky, long-term decisions in a constantly changing world.

This article describes home care information systems and their standard features. It also discusses the development process and issues raised as home care agencies move into the information age.

[Haworth co-indexing entry note]: "Home Health Care Information Systems: Difficult Choices in Uncertain Times." Schoech, Dick, Janet Neff, and Karen Roberts. Co-published simultaneously in *Journal of Gerontological Social Work* (The Haworth Press, Inc.) Vol. 24, No. 3/4, 1995, pp. 95-115; and: *New Developments in Home Care Services for the Elderly: Innovations in Policy, Program, and Practice* (ed: Lenard W. Kaye) The Haworth Press, Inc., 1995, pp. 95-115. Single or multiple copies of this article are available from The Haworth Document Delivery Service [1-800-342-9678, 9:00 a.m. - 5:00 p.m. (EST)].

© 1995 by The Haworth Press, Inc. All rights reserved.

DEFINITION AND PERSPECTIVES

Definition

An information system consists of the following components:

- *People*–those who collect, store, retrieve, manipulate, and communicate information, for example, a bookkeeper.
- *Information*–characters, numbers, text, symbols, graphics, pictures, voice, animation, and video that denote meaning, such as the number of hours worked, the monthly salary of employees, or a picture of an employee.
- *Tools*–instruments and mechanisms to help accomplish a task, for example, a copy machine, a computer, or database management software. Systems are often identified by their tools. For example, busses are often seen as a mass transit system or a computer or data base management system is often seen as an agency information system.
- *Structures and methods*–entities and their relationships and the processes for data manipulation, for example, fund accounting concepts or the procedures a bookkeeper follows when writing a payroll check.
- *Documentation*–descriptions of a system and directions on how the system works, for example, an operator's manual or interactive help in software.

A *home care information system* is a system of people, procedures and equipment that collects, stores, retrieves, manipulates, and communicates information to support a home care program. The word system implies that organized and integrated processes manipulate the information to reach a user defined goal. Since different home care employees have different goals, the perception of a home care IS varies by the type of employee. To illustrate, two different perspectives on a home care IS are presented, that of an administrator and that of a field worker.

Home Health IS from the Perspective of Management

Managers must have information about their business in order to make sound business decisions. A Home Health information system needs to give managers and supervisors accurate and timely patient and statistical information. For example, a manager would want to know how many visits each discipline in a certain service area was making in order to analyze current staffing and plan for the future. In addition, a supervisor needs to be apprised of patient clinical information in order to supervise field staff adequately and make certain all regulations are followed. An information system would enable this data to be more readily available.

The above view of a home care IS typifies the responses to a survey of thirteen Baylor HomeCare managers who were asked: (1) What does a management information system mean to you in reference to home care? and (2) What do you need from a management information system? The common thread in the six responses to the survey related to easy and accurate access to patient information and the ability to interface all offices (some up to 120 miles away). The most frequent responses were:

- ability to track information, for example, all scheduled visits were performed and turned in, or all physician orders were sent and received;
- tabulation of data for quality improvement/quality assurance, for example, from basic census or patient roster reports, to productivity of staff reports, to length of visits, etc.;
- access to a clinical picture of the patient for supervisory assistance and also for insurance case management reporting;
- management reports that easily assist one in identifying problems and trends; and
- minimal or no duplication of data entry.

Home Health IS from the Perspective of the Field

Most field staff welcome a good IS. They want a system that is easy to use and provides them with quick access to information they currently cannot obtain from the field. For example, an on-call nurse may need to confirm that a patient is currently on service. Even more important is a system that reduces the amount of time spent on paperwork and reduces the duplication of tasks involved in the sharing of information. For example, field staff would like an IS that quickly disseminates information to all who need it and eliminates the need for additional paperwork and phone calls.

The above view of a home care IS description typifies the responses to a survey of 60 Baylor HomeCare field staff (nurses, physical and speech therapists, and social workers) concerning what they needed from a computerized IS. Nineteen surveys were returned with at least two from each discipline. Some team members already had laptop computers, but most did not.

The survey found that staff wanted to send all their visit reports through the system as well as their schedules, discharge summaries, the plan of care and medical update (Health Care Financing Administration [HCFA] forms 485 and 486), changes in patients' status, recertifications, and revisit instructions. Staff wanted to be able to retrieve this same information, the information from the initial referral on the patient, and the schedules of other staff. Physician name, address and orders, lab results, and information about the activity of other services were also sought. Social workers wanted the patients' general demographics, diagnosis, income information, and services the patient was receiving.

LITERATURE REVIEW

Little has been written on the use of ISs for home care. Most literature is from professional trade magazines rather than journals.

Bergman (1993) reported on the use of computers by an HMO clinic to make "house calls" to patients. About 150 Boston area households used home computers as an interactive system through which the patients shared symptom information and answered a series of questions. Patients then received instructions about topics ranging from following self-care plans to going to the emergency room. Ninety percent of the patients were satisfied with the computer system. Bergman cited another study that concluded that the use of interactive computer programs in the home was a good method of early intervention with a potential for cost savings.

Minervino (1993) wrote about the use of computer systems to respond to the changes in the payment models for home care. Currently HCFA most frequently uses a *pay-per-visit* model that is based upon providers' existing costs. A *pay-per-episode* model is being tested that provides one payment for a single certification period (60 days). The payment is based on the patient's diagnosis and plan of care.

Minervino asserts that the success of a home care agency today is dependent upon the quality of its IS. Such systems must be flexible and able to respond quickly to changes in payment models. He identifies a good system as one that schedules nursing visits, allows for data entry of all clinical staff notes, identifies staff missing a case conference or team meeting, and identifies anything missing that a surveyor would look for on a chart. A good system would also include automated field devices, such as laptop computers, that allow for quick and accurate data entry. Minervino also emphasizes the need for good support services from the IS vendor.

Bailey and Dickson (1993) focused on the requirements of a home care IS in their 1988 study of home care nurses and the use of computers. The study showed that documentation and patient assessment were the activities that benefited most from a clinical computer system. Patient/family education and treatment/procedures also showed promised benefit from a computer system.

Bailey and Dickson identified the three major operational problems facing a home care agency as access to patient information, communication among the home care team, and time spent on documentation. The document requiring the most time was the treatment plan, followed by the nursing database, recertification, discharge documentation, and the HCFA 486 updates. The results of Bailey and Dickson's 1988 study indicated that a computer system would need to support documentation, patient assessment, treatment plans, and patient/family teaching activities.

Other features of a system discussed by Bailey and Dickson were:

- the information must be accessible 24 hours a day from a variety of locations;
- laptop PC's must contain a modem for easy loading and unloading of information;
- the system must be user friendly, that is, requiring a minimum of typing, utilization of simple windows with point and click menu and bar codes imputs, and templates of frequently used documentation available on an electronic clipboard;

- the system must be easy to carry and set up; and
- security is a critical consideration as is the accuracy, timeliness, and usability of the information.

FEATURES OF A HOME CARE INFORMATION SYSTEM

Features

A home care IS can consist of various groups of functions, depending on its complexity. For example, it can consist of intake, managed care, personnel, clinical, medical records, quality assurance, and billing (see Figure 1). The functions/features in Figure 1 are in-depth, but not all inclusive. When the functions/features of Figure 1 are used in a request for proposal (RFP), vendors would indicate whether each could be demonstrated at a client site, or is under development with a release date.

Expected Benefits

Each group of functions in Figure 1 has expected benefits. The expected benefits of the two major subsystems, billing and clinical, are presented.

A typical home care billing system has the following expected benefits:

- Improved timeliness and efficiency of departmental processing through the ability to locate and retrieve patient clinical and billing data.
- Improve patient care through the timely delivery of result reports to all areas.
- Improved patient processing and increased resource utilization through scheduling.
- Reduced lost charges due to unaccounted supplies and services through inventory management and control.
- Quicker turnaround of private and insurance billing and payments through the use of electronic data transfer.
- Better management control through productivity reporting, statistical manipulation, and consolidated financial reporting.

- Improved intake functionality by identifying prospective patients, better communications with other departments, and enhanced authorization and certification procedures.
- Improved medical records documentation and tracking mechanisms.
- Better communication of data among the various agencies, departments, branches, and affiliates.

A typical home care clinical system has the following expected benefits:

- System integration from the intake process to the final process of billing.
- Remote access to all patient information.
- Improved and more efficient data entry of visits due to on-line scheduling and entry of visits (i.e., remote laptop for clinician).
- Support of user defined care mapping, care planning, or outcomes management.
- Ability to produce and track all plans of care and verbal orders sent to physicians.
- Integrated ICD 9 (International Classification of Diseases, 9th Revision) coding package.
- Integrated word processing capabilities.
- Improved efficiency and increased time spent with patients by decreasing time on paperwork (i.e., point of care entry, minimal or non duplication of entry, error checking).

DEVELOPING INFORMATION SYSTEMS

The Development Process

Developing an information system requires planning, time, and effort as illustrated by the eight-step process presented in Figure 2. Buying commercial software or hiring information system expertise may bypass some tasks in each step of Figure 2, especially in the detailed design step. However, all tasks must be completed and

FIGURE 1. RFP example criteria for a home health care system.

General application requirements

Accesses patient data by patient's name or portion thereof?

Defines patient data purge criteria based on patient type, discharge/expire date, number of days of inactivity?

Has remote terminal access (dial-up) capabilities?

Prints reports to the screen?

Reprints any recently printed document?

Routes reports to multiple printers?

Sends and receives electronic mail messages among users?

Allows for correcting erroneously merged patient records?

Entry/update of patient medical and billing data is made on-line and takes effect immediately, such that the next person to access the data gets the most current data entered?

System can monitor usage such as disk space, file size, etc.?

In the event of any system failure, automatically recover all files to the last completed transactions, and notify users of any incomplete transactions not recovered when normal operations resume?

Data entry devices are secured against unauthorized use?

Provide a two level sign-on function composed of user ID and a user modifiable password?

Logs unauthorized access attempts by terminal, date, and time?

Can automatically log user off the system if there is no activity within a user-specified period of time?

Shows the date and production time on all printed documents?

Report writer can produce ad-hoc reports?

Provides multiple security controls based upon user sign-on and/or terminal ID?

Password security can be defined at the field level for each user as read, add, change, and delete?

Provide on-line help function usable without interrupting the data entry or other processes?

Supports field highlightings, blinking, standard characters, and reverse video display, as well as color terminals?

Supports keyboard or type-ahead buffers allowing fast data entry?

Upload and download data to and from a microcomputer?

All screens have sufficient prompts so as to be self-explanatory? When a choice of action is possible, all commands are presented to the user to allow selection?

Intake requirements/managed care

Interfaces with other home care departments?

Can allow more than one physician to be added to the patient information?

If the patient is rehospitalized with home care, can obtain previous history and current orders?

Assigns Medicare ICD-9 code to patient diagnosis using a search feature?

Provides statistical information such as: referral sources, number of evaluations in a month, number of evaluations requested, etc.

Automatically discharges patients who have been hospitalized more than a set number of days?

Generates a report of patients who have not been admitted to the system within 30 days from the preadmit date for verification?

Case manager or insurance company contact person can be entered on admission, along with any negotiated prices, phone numbers, and addresses?

Generates a letter to case manager on negotiated price?

Allows referral information to be edited daily?

Preschedules patient with name and potential start-of-care date and routes to skilled nursing, physical therapy, home health aide, medical social work and private duty? Can a daily report of this information be generated?

Has readmit capability?

Allows input of hourly rate as well as a per visit rate?

Produces reports and graphs regarding number of referrals by physician per month; number of admits per month; number of nonadmits per months/rationale; number of visits made in PM, weekends, holidays; and number of referrals by physician specialty or illness?

Tracks revenue produced per office (affiliates and branches)?

Tracks number of referrals by insurance class?

Provides reports with concurrent information on costs versus anticipated reimbursement for contract covered patients?

Provides an analysis report of HMO/PPO performance relative to contract?

Analyzes utilization patterns by type of therapy, demographics, and physician?

Personnel management requirements

Stores employee masterfile information?

Tracks applicant information?

Tracks licensure and continuing education to insure requirements have been met?

Does integrated payroll?

FIGURE 1 (continued)

Clinical requirements

System allows for remote, point of service, entry of data?

System generates all needed paperwork and forms for home care agency?

Remote devices allow for 2-way communication: (1) download of patient information into the data entry device from a host or central storage, (2) load updated information back to the host or central storage?

Clinical information system interfaces directly with the home care billing system?

HCFA acceptable electronic signatures for notes and forms are supported by the system?

Clinical information system utilizes codified data entry methods to enable quick, nontext entry, as well as meaningful data analysis?

The system has the capability to access patient records from a repository of patient information that contains hospital, physician office, and other clinical data?

System is capable of maintaining schedules for all field staff?

The system allows either the supervisor/scheduler or the case manager to enter their own schedule?

The schedule system allows an area for type of visit reason, an area for nonadmits, and reason for nonadmission?

The system has a feature whereby every visit scheduled is accounted for when documentation is received?

The clinical information system supports user-defined care maps? (Care maps include the plan of care as well as comparison of actual outcomes to the plans.)

The system produces HCFA forms 485/86s in draft format allowing supervisory review and correction directly into the system to be edited by authorized personnel?

The system reprints any verbal order by physician or patient?

The system tracks the status of all verbal orders?

The system updates the medication sheet automatically based on verbal orders related to medication changes?

The system flags if all orders have been carried out at time of discharge?

The system incorporates an integrated word processing package for transcription?

The system generates management reports regarding:
- Staff's productivity per clinician
- Staff's documentation problems per clinician
- Staff's mileage per clinician, and
- Staff's patient care problems (observation from home visits)?

The system generates a discharge summary automatically after the last skilled visit, allowing information to be added or changed on line?

Medical records requirements

Has a returned/mailed report for standard home care HCFA form 485?

Has an outstanding verbal orders tickler?

Reprints previous periods for HCFA forms 485/486/487?

Reprints verbal orders by physician or patient?

Produces a recertifications due and overdue list?

Has admission and discharge tracking? Can generate a list of admission and discharge paperwork that is incomplete?

Allows for discharges by one discipline and/or one agency?

Has rehospitalized tracking?

Quality assurance requirements

Generates labels for all addresses (MD/patient/employees/payors)?

Generates physician utilization reports?

Generates a list of patients by length of stay?

Generates a list of patients by ICD-9 codes?

Generates a list of rehospitalized patients by month?

Generates discharges by one discipline?

Has rehospitalized tracking and tickler system?

Has on-hold tracking and tickler system?

Prints outstanding claims by month?

Produces census by location/branch or discipline?

Produces unpaid claims details with reason and location/branch?

Can individual screens be developed to capture infection rates, QA data, etc., and automatically calculate percentage rates?

Allows user-defined fields for specialized, customized reporting without vendor intervention?

Allows user to edit verbal orders and reprint?

Billing requirements

Transfers billing data from one funding source or institution to another if error is found?

Prints HCFA 1500 forms as well as the UB-92 form?

Can override on form locators for insurance companies and workers' compensation claims?

Can leave form locators blank on UB-92 form as well as HCFA forms 485, 486 and 487.

Accesses previously entered visits to add supplies or make changes?

Enters all adjustments (price, reason, etc.) and generates a hard copy for signature and then updates the A/R?

FIGURE 1 (continued)

Allows for on-line input of account notes for each patient account and denial management?

Produces an end-of-month report that reflects closing statistics?

Can issue split bills?

Can reprint a bill?

Generates a deposit log after payments are posted?

Pulls up and prints bills for all funding sources and branches at the same time? If so, can other users still put information into the system?

Retains old price when price is updated for late charge purposes on visits?

Runs late billing for multiple months, financial classes and institutions?

Can user hold production of bill until all established criteria is met (ICD-9 codes/485 complete, etc.)?

Generates an edit of all bills pending for lack of information and description of missing information?

Accommodates flags on uncredentialed physicians?

Electronic Media Claims (EMC) approved by intermediary?

Can change the supply/visit price for unbilled supplies/visits for current month?

User enters multiple visits/supplies by selecting what dates are needed?

Can do "visit entry" and "supply entry" on the same screen?

Records supply inventory on hand, supplies withdrawn from inventory by RN's, and supplies used by each individual?

Runs supply lists by branch/office?

Accommodates bar-coding of supplies?

Makes provisions for Medicare nonbillable supplies?

Allows for mass price changes (percentage increases)?

Multiple entry of charges for financial class and institution can be established?

Changes Medicare supply to or from nonbill status?

Safety feature prevents established supply codes from being duplicated to another branch/office?

Prices by box and by unit without having to code supply twice?

FIGURE 2. The process of information system development.

Step 1: Assess Preparedness and Feasibility
  Communicate about the IS effort to all staff.
  Establish a steering committee.
  Define the IS purpose, objectives, development timetables, and responsibilities.
  Estimate resources for change, i.e., money, time, expertise, commitment of key individuals.
  Estimate improved system impacts (positive & negative).
  Assess the expectations and reactions of those who will be affected by the IS.
  Prepare and circulate preparedness and feasibility report.
  Decide to proceed or terminate effort.

Step 2: Analysis of Existing System (Systems Analysis)
  Identify the major tasks and decisions the IS will support and the information needed to support them.
  Define the characteristics of the information needed, its source, and collection methods.
  Analyze current and future data input, processing, and output operations and requirements, e.g., forms, manipulations, files, and reports.
  Describe logical routing or flow of information from collection to dissemination.
  Evaluate problems with the existing IS.
  Review similar efforts in other agencies and request help from national or state associations.
  Prepare and circulate systems analysis report.
  Decide to proceed or terminate effort.

Step 3: Conceptual Design
  Finalize IS scope, goals, and objectives.
  Develop alternative conceptual designs, i.e., fields, records, files, data manipulation, forms, and reports.
  Apply restrictions to potential designs, i.e., required and desired data frequency, volume, security, confidentiality, turn around time; and IS flexibility, reliability, processing and statistical capabilities, growth potential, life expectancy, and tie-in with other systems.
  Apply resources to designs, e.g., money, time, and expertise.
  Translate designs into software and hardware configurations.
  Detail the advantages, disadvantages and assumptions of alternate designs.
  Prepare and circulate conceptual design and decide to proceed or terminate effort.

Step 4: Detailed Design and Development
  Set up controls and technical performance standards for chosen design.
  Select the software for the chosen design.
  Select the hardware to accommodate the software.
  Design and develop input forms, data manipulations, processing operations, file specifications, database structures, indexes, error checks, storage and backup mechanisms and procedures, and output reports.
  Prepare programming documentation and instruction manuals.

Step 5: System Testing and Agency Preparation
  Prepare system operators, users, and others to receive the system.
  Develop agency policy and procedural changes necessary for the new system.
  Develop performance criteria and testing plan.

FIGURE 2 (continued)

Test programming, forms, operational procedures, instructions, reports, and the use of outputs.
Educate and train system operators, data users, and others affected.

Step 6: Conversion
Develop and approve conversion plan, for example, stop old system when new system starts or run old and new systems simultaneously for comparison.
Incorporate IS into standard operating procedures, for example, performance appraisals, new employee orientation.
Reorganize staff and space if necessary.
Convert from old to new equipment, new processing methods, and new procedures.
Insure all systems and controls are working.

Step 7: Evaluation
Compare system performance with initial system objectives, e.g., if system improved client services.
Relate benefits and costs to initial estimates.
Measure satisfaction with the system.
Determine if system outputs are used in decision making.

Step 8: Operation, Maintenance and Modification
Prepare backup and emergency plans and procedures.
Complete documentation, e.g., instructions for adding to, deleting from, or modifying system.
Assign persons responsible for data integrity, system maintenance, new software appropriateness, virus protection, etc.
Provide continuous training of users.
Continue to add desired enhancements and to maintain and debug the system.
Begin step 1 if additional subsystems are to be developed.

- - - - - - - - - - - - - -

Note: From "Strategies for Information System Development," by D. Schoech, L. L. Schkade, & R. S. Mayers. (1982). *Administration in Social Work, 5*(3/4), 25-26. Copyright 1981 by The Haworth Press, Inc. Adapted by permission.

documented somewhere. Some steps are completed by the vendor before a product goes to market.

The information system development process is iterative. Each step builds on and amplifies activities of the previous step. For example, the first step, assessing preparedness and feasibility, must be given repeated consideration throughout the process. Although the IS development process may appear to be a precise science, at present it is more of an art.

The development of an IS depends on many factors, such as agency power structure and the ease of programming a solution to the chosen problems. Consequently, systems developed are often those that serve management needs or are most feasible rather than those that are most needed.

Accompanying Organizational Changes

Successful ISs require preparation, planning, commitment, and involvement. Each subsystem should be part of a total agency IS plan. Top management must show commitment by guiding the overall effort and placing IS development function in a separate, high level department. Management must also insure that representatives of users and others affected serve on an IS development committee and keep their constituents informed and involved throughout the process.

Developing an information system should be a gradual process. One module should be implemented at a time, and the total process should be well documented. Continuity of system developers should be assured. However, this may be difficult with the scarcity and mobility of well-trained staff.

A rule for developing successful information systems is to spend 10 percent of total resources on hardware, 40 percent on software and software development, and 50 percent on implementation and training. With current fiscal constraints, many fail to budget adequately for the 50 percent associated with implementation and training.

ISSUES

Source of the Home Care IS

Perhaps the biggest IS decision for a home care agency is how to proceed with development. ISs may be purchased from a vendor or custom built by a home care provider. Vendor systems are generic and may be difficult to adapt to local needs. Due to frequent changes in hardware, software, and the home care field, the viability and farsightedness of the vendor become crucial in keeping the software current.

In choosing a vendor, home care agencies must decide whether to purchase from a general health care vendor that has a home care subsystem, or from a vendor that specializes in home care. The advantage of a general health care vendor is that the vendor is large and the home care IS purchased will probably interface well with the larger system. The disadvantage is that the general health care vendor may not see home care as their specialty and fail to give the home care IS the attention and resources required to develop and maintain a high quality home care system. Purchasing from a vendor who specializes in home care may provide a more tailored IS, but interface with the larger health care system could be a problem. Also, we are in an age of mergers and acquisitions. A home care vendor may be purchased by a generic health care vendor that views the home care IS product differently and is not committed to maintaining a high quality product.

Another difficult choice is whether to go with an innovative vendor that often has the latest technology or with a vendor with a longtime track record that is often wedded to older technology. Vendor stability and performance is probably the wisest choice over the long run, although vendor stability is difficult to determine. A beginning list of vendors appears in Figure 3. Being on the list does not represent an endorsement of the vendor's product.

If agencies custom build their own IS, cost, technical expertise, maintenance, and future changes become crucial issues. While a

FIGURE 3. Sample list of vendors.

Vendor	Phone number
Atlantic West Services	412-439-2933
Comprehensive Health Systems	305-599-9992
Delta Computer Systems	814-944-1651
Home Care Information Systems	201-338-2020
Lewis Computer Services	504-927-3065
Management Software Incorporated	417-883-2900
Smart Clipboard Corporation	314-993-0665

custom built system may be better adapted to agency needs, it can be costly and quickly become outdated. Commercial vendors pay for the high cost of software development and maintenance by mass sales. Agencies that custom build software must bear the cost alone or continually lag behind. Home care agencies should evaluate system costs over the long run before developing their own system. The initial cost/benefit calculations for custom built ISs may seem attractive, but typically systems are over budget and behind schedule. However, the real problem with custom built systems is continued maintenance and enhancements. In a stable marketplace, developing a custom system makes sense. However, stability is lacking in hardware, software, and especially the home care industry. Given this change, the life of a home care system may be 1.5 to two years before substantial revisions must be made. Often custom systems need to be redesigned as soon as they are completed. Consequently, custom developed systems often stagnate due to personnel changes, budget cuts, and lack of energy.

Interface with the Larger Systems

Systems theory predicts that one of the most problematic areas of an information system is its interface with other systems (Schoech, 1990). This is especially true of the interface of a home care IS with the larger health system of which it is a part. With home care being one of the newest health care areas, standardization rarely exists. Often, the vendor that supplies the IS to the larger system views home care differently than the home care agency.

The reverse is also true. If a home care provider finds an IS that fits its needs well, the IS may not interface well with the larger system. For example, a hospital based home care agency may not be able to interface their home care system with the hospital admission or discharge system.

Impact of Low Income and Source of Funds on the IS Selection

Several special considerations are necessary for home care ISs that serve low income clients. The IS will need to identify funding sources that often dictate the type and amount of services a patient receives. Medicare covers nursing, social work, home health aides, physical, speech, and occupational therapy, and allows as many visits as needed with adequate documentation. Medicaid is more limiting of the number of visits a patient receives per year and does not reimburse for social work. Medicaid patients are often among the most in need of social work services. Other patients will be in managed care or capitated plans, or have no coverage at all. It will be necessary for all team members to be aware of the patient's payment source (or sources) and the parameters associated with this plan. It is also helpful for the IS to provide the general economic status of patients. This information will alert the home care team to concerns related to cost of medications, medical equipment and supplies not covered by insurance, and the cost of outside help for the patient's care.

Access, Security, Confidentiality, and Privacy

One persistent set of issues concerns information access, security, confidentiality, and privacy (Schoech, 1990).

Access concerns who has rights to the information collected and generated when serving clients. Access is becoming increasingly important due to information technology and health care reform. Health care reform seems to be placing more responsibility for quality health care on patients who now have the technology to store and synthesize personal health information. Consequently, we must consider what access and control over health information belong to the home care provider, the client, the insurance industry, or other participants such as legal guardians. For example, do clients or client advocacy groups have legal access to agency information that does not identify individual clients for purposes such as establishing trends in services or in malpractice?

Security involves the physical protection of information using locks and other barriers. With proper security, a person may be allowed to read, but not to change or delete certain parts of a client record. As Bailey and Dickson (1993) point out, security becomes a more salient concern when field staff begin using laptop computers from numerous locations.

Confidentiality concerns the agreed level of restriction placed on information by the practitioner and the client. As more databases are linked, security and confidentiality become a challenge for hardware and software technicians, agency policy, and the policy of the total health care system. Confidentiality becomes more difficult as an increased amount of information becomes available to more and more users in a variety of places including patients' homes and the homes of field staff. Often it is difficult for the home care professional to promise confidentiality when they have no control over the use of client information by others involved such as employers, employee assistance programs, or managed care companies. It is difficult for home care professionals to adequately inform their clients regarding confidentiality since this area is still evolving.

Privacy concerns a client's right to keep personal information secret. For example, can the client withhold information not essential for service delivery? Or, can clients receive services if they refuse to allow their information to be stored in a home care IS?

While the above issues are important, the most difficult issues in IS development concerns handling the rapid and pervasive changes associated with ISs, for example, resistance, effective use, and job restructuring. The key issue involves how to manage the people change associated with technological change.

SPECIAL CONSIDERATIONS
DUE TO HEALTH CARE REFORM

The environment of health care is in the state described by Emery and Trist (1965) as a "turbulent field." This is a dynamic condition in which changes arise from the field itself. "The 'ground' is in motion" (p. 27) is a phrase that describes a turbulent field. This turbulent field results when the interdependence between economic conditions and other aspects of society increase and when organizations become more involved in regulation and legislation. Health care is changing from a physician driven model to one influenced by a broad scope of directors including payers, health care systems, and the government. At the present, little is certain about the composition of the final system.

Another change involves how home care is offered in insurance plans. One possibility is home care being offered as part of a long-term health plan. In the past the only long-term health plan option was a nursing home. Now, insurance plans may open up a whole new market and future for home care.

A final change that is occurring, in one form or another, is prospective payment. The home care industry, that has been cost reimbursed for the past 10 years, is largely shifting to a prospective pay system. Predictions about prospective payment range from a totally capitated system, to a DRG type system, or to a form of co-payment type system. Medicare/Medicaid reimbursement and private insurance reimbursement will probably look much more similar than in the past.

As the health care model moves from "pay per visit" to "payment by diagnosis," a computer system will need to monitor information about patient needs and the expenses incurred in providing patient care. The system will need to incorporate means of efficiently improving patient care such as care mapping and outcome measures. Additionally, the system will need to facilitate communication among medical team members, billing personnel, supply clerks, and managers. The system will need the capacity to interface with the larger system with which the agency is affiliated, especially hospitals, rehabilitation facilities, and even physician offices. A comprehensive computer IS will be an essential tool in meeting the demands of providing health care in the future.

Minervino (1993) addressed the role of technology in health care reform as he emphasized the necessity of a flexible and comprehensive IS. Cutting cost while maintaining quality care is the chief goal of health care reform and becomes the primary goal of a home care IS. Lower costs are to be achieved by enabling field and administrative staff to save time through use of the IS. The system must also be able to change rapidly to accommodate changes in computerized billing systems and documentation requirements.

The above trends and special considerations challenge a home care IS to interface with current systems from hospital to physician offices in order to keep costs down and quality consistent. According to Shay Fields (personal communication, August 10, 1994), Administrative Director for Baylor HomeCare, "Cost accounting is going to be crucial ... it will be imperative that an agency knows its costs, they cannot afford to operate in a vacuum." Efficiency and accuracy will also be crucial. While reimbursement may decrease in the above models, the cost of running the agency will remain constant or increase. Automating an agency will be crucial. These rapid environmental changes also suggest home care agencies should not develop their own IS but rely on a vendor capable of keeping their software current with reforms.

CONCLUSION

Developing an IS requires definition, standardization, and specification. Given the newness of home care as a health care subsystem and the rapid changes due to health care reform and managed care, IS development involves some very difficult and risky decisions. The goal is to know your internal and external data needs and choose a vendor that is up-to-date, yet stable. A vendor that specializes in home care, yet understands the larger system, is desirable. Documenting needs and finding such a vendor is difficult given the limited resources many home care agencies have to devote to IS development. A fair summary of the current situation is that home care ISs are difficult to develop and maintain, but impossible to do without.

REFERENCES

Bailey, J. and Dickson, N. (1993). "Analyzing home care information system needs," *Caring Magazine*, 12, 34-37.
Bergman, R. (1993). "Computers make 'house calls' to patients," *Hospitals*, 67, 52.
Emery, F. E. and Trist, E. L. (1965). "The causal texture of organizational environments," *Human Relations*, 18, 21-32.
Minervino, M. (1993). "Efficiency with software information systems under prospective pay," *Caring Magazine*, 12, 46-51.
Schoech, D. (1990). *Human services computing: Concepts and applications*. New York, NY: The Haworth Press, Inc.

Chapter 6

Evaluation and Quality Assurance
for In-Home Services

Susan L. Hughes, DSW

The capacity to conduct internal evaluations can be both a strategic asset and a competitive advantage for home care programs. Evaluation research is unique among the social sciences in that it involves the direct application of research techniques to practical problems associated with the delivery of services. In essence, evaluations seek to determine how and why programs work (process) and how and whether program processes impact outcomes. Thus, evaluations are very "hands on" and very much concerned with the nuts and bolts of how specific programs work.

Evaluations can vary greatly with respect to their foci and methods. In general, three broad classes of evaluations exist, namely; formative evaluations, process or program evaluations, and summative or outcome evaluations. Each of these types or "models" is useful for particular types of issues under specific conditions. This chapter illustrates the use of these methods for different types of problems and at different levels of the home care agency–e.g., the administrator, the staff, and program clients. It also illustrates how evaluation tools can be applied in implementing new quality assurance methods like Continuous Quality Improvement and Total

[Haworth co-indexing entry note]: "Evaluation and Quality Assurance for In-Home Services." Hughes, Susan L. Co-published simultaneously in *Journal of Gerontological Social Work* (The Haworth Press, Inc.) Vol. 24, No. 3/4, 1995, pp. 117-131; and: *New Developments in Home Care Services for the Elderly: Innovations in Policy, Program, and Practice* (ed: Lenard W. Kaye) The Haworth Press, Inc., 1995, pp. 117-131. Single or multiple copies of this article are available from The Haworth Document Delivery Service [1-800-342-9678, 9:00 a.m. - 5:00 p.m. (EST)].

© 1995 by The Haworth Press, Inc. All rights reserved.   *117*

Quality Management. Finally, the chapter concludes with thoughts about human resources needed to conduct these studies and the types of data and data processing that can be required.

FORMATIVE EVALUATIONS

Formative evaluations are generally most appropriate when an agency is considering adopting a new service line about which little information currently exists. For example, an agency might be considering the initiation of a special "wake-up" or "tuck-in" service for clients. As a first step, staff with responsibility for planning the service could review existing literature or other agencies' experience with this service. Simultaneously, staff could survey a sample of active clients to determine their degree of interest in the service and convene separate focus groups of clients, agency staff, and referral sources to estimate demand, staffing needs, costs, and willingness to pay for these new types of care.

A second step could involve implementing the service on a pilot basis with a small sample of clients, along with a telephone survey of client satisfaction, the results of which could be used to "debug" the service and iron out kinks in service delivery from the client's perspective. Finally, once these steps have been implemented the agency could consider, based on its experience, whether it makes sense to proceed with full-scale, agency or catchment area wide implementation of the new service.

As this example of a relatively simple service innovation indicates, formative evaluations can be used as an aid to sound strategic planning. In order to succeed, the evaluation process should involve representatives from all the different groups (stakeholders) that need to be involved in the new service, including administrative, billing, referral sources, clinical staff, and clients and families. Although the example given here is purposely a simple one, similar kinds of steps can be taken to evaluate more complex service initiatives such as the development/acquisition of a high tech home care product line. Generally speaking, the more complex and technologically sophisticated the new initiative is, the greater the number of stakeholders who will need to be drawn into active participation in the planning/evaluation process.

PROCESS EVALUATIONS

As the name implies, a process evaluation examines the implementation of a given service in order to increase efficiency, productivity, effectiveness, and/or consider whether a particular service should be dropped from the agency's portfolio. Process evaluations are very similar to operations research and are used frequently for continuous quality improvement (CQI). In contrast to quality assurance (QA), which attempts to ensure that care meets some minimal standard, CQI attempts to achieve excellence by continually examining and improving/fine-tuning the processes of care (Berwick, 1989).

CQI assumes that everyone in the agency is trying to do a good job but that service systems or operations can benefit from scrutiny if they are to meet or exceed the needs and expectations of consumers. Take, for example, staff in a hospital-linked home health care agency who observe a large number of inappropriate referrals or number of cases that do not receive recertification by a physician in a timely way. The VNA in Chicago (VNAC) experienced this situation working with the University of Chicago Hospitals (UCH) with whom it had a preferred provider contract (Leimnetzer, Ryan, and Niemann, 1993). It became apparent to staff at both providers that successful implementation of care required formal methods of sharing information. To achieve this goal, senior level staff in both agencies were identified to guide the development of a formal coordination process. As a first step in this process the VNA set up a separate CQI program specifically for UCH patients. Next, staff reviewed steps involved in referrals, intake, patient-nurse assignment and initial start of care processes. This review found that most start of care delays were caused by inaccurate demographic information and by reception of final orders on the last day of hospitalization as opposed to the day before. As a result of the review, both agencies agreed to a new set of ground rules. The hospital notifies VNAC of pending discharges but holds the referral until final orders are received, the UCH discharge planning staff make special efforts to verify patients' destination at discharge, and both parties agreed to formal criteria for prioritizing patient assignment based on acuity level. Simultaneously, one-on-one interviews were held with representatives of five different practitioner groups involved in coordinating patients' care. Through this process it was possible to achieve consensus across disciplines that the physician would be designated as the primary contact for feedback. These clarifications in program operations greatly enhanced the efficiency and continuity of patient care.

According to Bobnet et al. (1993), several conditions need to be met in order to implement a CQI program in a home care agency. First, top management (including the Board of Directors) must commit to the need for CQI and the concepts that guide it. Second, an upper management resource group that represents all key areas of the organization (clinical, financial, personnel, and information systems) needs to be identified. This group educates itself about CQI, and develops the quality vision, quality policy and quality values of the organization. Finally, this group develops policy and procedures for the CQI process.

The next step involves the creation of CQI teams to evaluate specific agency processes and make improvements over time. The resource group can review staff requests for the establishment of specific teams to prevent duplication of effort. Teams should be small (six to 10 members) and include representation of all groups involved in the process being studied. Both a team leader and a facilitator should be designated. The facilitator can be a member of the resource group. Meetings should be limited to one hour per month with subgroup meetings as necessary. Team progress reports should be as simple as possible, with minutes submitted quarterly to the CQI coordinator. Progress should ultimately be shared with the entire organization through the minutes and through an internal newsletter.

The implementation of a meaningful, well-functioning CQI capacity can take as long as five years to complete. However, once implementation is complete, the process accelerates as CQI teams become a part of daily program activities. At this stage, the resource group no longer needs to closely supervise the teams but can truly act in a resource capacity. Although the implementation of CQI requires substantial investment in process evaluation by agencies, agencies which have implemented it believe it is very effective in ensuring internal and external customer and staff satisfaction, thus providing an important competitive advantage.

OUTCOME OR SUMMATIVE EVALUATIONS

As the name implies, outcome evaluations attempt to learn whether programs make a difference in impacting some outcome of interest. As a general rule, outcome evaluations should be reserved for a time when the intervention or program is well-established, when program staff have a good idea about who the appropriate target population is and know how to successfully enroll that population. In addition, it is important that the new program has had a test run during which service has been debugged and fine-tuned. Finally, it is critically important that program staff articulate why and how a specific new service is expected to impact a specific outcome for the specific population to whom the service is targeted.

Although outcome evaluations are recommended only for programs that have reached a mature state, home care was subjected to outcome studies very early while still a new service modality. This concentration on outcomes reflects policymakers' concerns regarding home care cost effectiveness. Given the rapid growth in home care programs, clients, and expenditures, policymakers wanted to know how home care impacts total health care costs. In turn, providers somewhat rashly promised cost-savings that could be achieved by substituting home care for costly institutional care. As a result of premature but understandably zealous pursuit of evidence showing an impact on cost, policymakers, providers, and evaluators rushed to conduct summative evaluations, before articulating theories about how these new services could be expected to work and why. As a result we have experienced 25-30 years of summative evaluations that have produced very contradictory findings concerning effectiveness (Hughes, 1985; Hedrick and Inui, 1986; Kemper et al., 1988a; Weissert, Cready and Pawelak, 1988).

In my view, the conflicting research findings to date largely reflect the lack of a coherent theoretical approach to the study of home care. Take, for example, the National Long Term Care Demonstration. This multi-site demonstration was intended to provide an unequivocal answer to the "substitution" question. In other words this study was supposed to determine whether case managed community care saved money by substituting home/community-based long term care for more expensive hospital or nursing home care (Kemper et al., 1988b).

Unfortunately, however, people who designed the evaluation did not spend enough time thinking through in advance exactly how and why chanelling would impact hospital and nursing home use. If they had developed a "logic model" spelling out how the intervention would work before implementing the evaluation they would have realized something very important–specifically, nurses and social work case management teams do not make decisions to hospitalize or institutionalize people. Rather, these decisions are made by patients, patients' families, and physicians. Thus, a community-based intervention that consists of a nurse/social work team is not likely to impact hospital or nursing home use. And, in fact, that is what the evaluation found. Specifically, although case management improved clients' satisfaction with care, reduced clients' unmet service needs, and made clients more confident that their needs would be met, it did not reduce hospital or nursing home admissions in the treatment group vis-à-vis the controls. Thus, the evaluation design and the intervention suffered from theory failure, e.g., inadequate specification of the method through which the new program would achieve its desired outcomes.

Other earlier evaluations of community-based care also suffered from conceptual flaws. For example, the Community Care Organization in Wisconsin attempted to test the impact of case management on people who were at high risk of nursing home admission. Since the state was mainly interested in reducing Medicaid nursing home expenditures, the demonstration was limited to clients in the community who were already Medicaid eligible. As a result, the demonstration targeted a young-old population that bears little resemblance to the typical nursing home population. The evaluators didn't realize that their *real* at-risk population was elderly and disabled people with poor social supports living in the community who were not receiving Medicaid but who would become Medicaid eligible after they spent down their resources during their first few months of nursing home use. Thus, in addition to having a defensible theory about how and why the program will work, it is also necessary to know what population should be targeted to receive the intervention.

Once these issues are clarified, many other issues remain. For example, it is important to be able to access the at-risk population in a systematic way. In some cases it may even be necessary for program staff to do their own casefinding. If casefinding is needed, a feasible method of conducting it–both in terms of funding and manpower–must be found.

Third, it also is important to obtain good process measures that can be examined to determine how well the intervention was implemented. Process measures can be used to demonstrate quantitatively whether the intervention involved a reasonable number of visits of a specific type. For example, one would not expect to see improvements in physical functioning among older home care clients unless the intervention has a high concentration of physical therapy or aides trained to provide some type of exercise intervention. Keeping tabs on the types of services used by clients in both the intervention and comparison groups is especially helpful when findings indicate no treatment effect. They enable us to assess whether the intervention was implemented well but had no effect or whether it was not implemented successfully. The steps taken to remedy the situation obviously would differ greatly, depending on one's interpretation of why no result was observed. In many cases, the properties of home care interventions have been described very sketchily in outcome evaluations and, only rarely, in quantifiable terms (Hughes, Cordray and Spiker, 1984).

Condition-specific outcome measures also help one to detect a treatment effect. Although this step is important it is not always simple to do because it implies that outcomes should be based on the characteristics of the targeted groups and what is known about the impact of those characteristics on outcomes of interest like health services utilization, functional status, and quality of life.

Finally, in addition to these conditions, decisions must be made about methods to be used. Although many home care evaluations use single group, before and after comparisons, the use of a comparison group is very important in preventing premature acceptance of program impact. In many cases, people improve on some outcome such as client satisfaction, simply because they are trying to please agency staff or because they are aware that they are being measured. The use of a comparison group, especially a randomly drawn comparison group, can help to rule out some of these plausible, rival explanations of treatment effects. It also is important to enroll samples that are large enough for the treatment to show an effect. Many randomized trials have failed to find an effect because they lacked statistical power–the sample tested was simply too small. A social psychologist or statistician in a local School of Public Health, Medical, Nursing and/or Social Work, can serve as an important consultant for this type of design issue.

Finally, assuming one has chosen a strong design with an appropriate size sample, it is very important to use reliable and valid pre- and posttest measures. Many valid generic quality of life and disease-specific outcome measures are available today with more and more coming on line (Kane and Kane, 1981, Ware and Sherburn, 1992). Again, a review of the literature and consultation with academics are invaluable aids to the selection of measures that are best for a specific study.

Some examples of summative evaluations of team-managed home care may help to illustrate these points. Several years ago we used a randomized experimental design to test the cost-effectiveness of team-managed hospital-based home care (TM/HBHC) in the VA. This study was initiated at the instigation of and in collaboration with the Medical Director of the Hines V.A. Hospital HBHC program. The Hines model was unique with respect to its ability to provide continuous team-managed home care, including physician care, within and outside the acute care setting. Hines HBHC staff believed that this model provided cost-effective care for two specific patient groups–those with two or more ADL impairments and the terminally ill. The outcome evaluation examined this issue by prospectively screening all acute admissions to the 1100-bed Hines facility over a three-year period to identify and randomize 233 severely disabled veteran and caregiver pairs and 171 terminally ill veteran and informal caregiver pairs to TM/HBHC or to customary care.

Findings included significant increases in patient and caregiver satisfaction with care that were accompanied by net cost savings of 10% in the severely disabled group and 18% in the terminally ill group, yielding a net cost savings of 13% (Hughes et al., 1990; Hughes et al., 1992; Cummings et al., 1990). Although this net cost savings was not statistically significant, it is the largest cost savings reported to date in the home care literature. Importantly, the savings were largely attributable to reductions in hospital readmission days. As a result, cost of readmission hospital care was 24% lower in the severely disabled intervention group and 39.5% lower in the terminally ill intervention group, yielding a significant hospital readmission cost savings of 29% (p = .03) for the two groups combined.

Although these findings suggest that this home care model has the potential to reduce cost of care while simultaneously increasing patient and caregiver satisfaction with care, a trial with substantially more patients and additional sites is necessary to definitively test the effect of the model on costs and to assess the model's generalizability in the VA. These issues are currently being addressed in a VA cooperative study of TM/HBHC. This study began on January 1, 1993 and involves replicating and testing the TM/HBHC model at 15 VA hospitals across the country with a sample of 2,900 patients (Cummings, Hughes and Weaver, 1992).

Because the generalizability of the model to the private health care sector is currently unknown, we have adapted this new home care model for use and testing in the private sector. We believe that TM/HBHC succeeded in the VA because it encourages physician involvement in managing patient care. Physicians in the VA have no financial incentive to retain patients in their practices because they are salaried. Therefore, it is possible for VA HBHC patients to be transferred from the admitting physician to the HBHC physician for ongoing care management inside and outside of the hospital. The HBHC physician does not routinely make home visits to active patients but is available to review patients with the home care team, to visit patients at home as necessary and to facilitate planned versus emergency patient readmissions.

Incentives for physician involvement in Medicare home health care are quite different. All referrals for Medicare home care emanate from a physician, but the physician's role in home care treatment is usually minimal. Frequently, a hospital discharge planner refers a patient to a home care provider at the physician's request. The home care staff visits the patient at home to confirm that the patient has a condition that is reimbursable by Medicare. If so, the home care agency fills out the physician patient care orders on the HCFA 485 Start of Care form and sends the form to the physician for signature.

After home care begins, the burden of provider/physician communication about the patient's condition is assumed by the home care provider. Medicare requires home health care providers to obtain physician recertification of the patient's continued need for care at 60 days following the start of care. However, little is known about the pattern and quality of communication that takes place between home care providers and the large number of physicians who can be responsible for patients receiving home care on any given day. In fact, until 1993, Medicare actually discouraged physician involvement in home care by setting payment for physician home visits at a lower rate than that of home health aides (Rust, 1992).

In response to this problem, the AMA has developed and disseminated generic physician home care practice guidelines. Some home care providers have hired medical directors to interface with referring physicians when necessary and to provide medical guidance for nursing staff. Although both of these developments are probably helpful, they may not be sufficient to ensure optimal patient care outcomes, given the increasing complexity and severity of medical conditions treated in the home.

In order to develop and test a TM/HLHC model for use in the private sector, we held extensive discussions with the administrators of Northwestern Memorial Home Health Care, Inc., the hospital-*linked* subsidiary which provides home health care services for patients discharged from our University affiliate, Northwestern Memorial Hospital. We discussed the features of the TM/HLHC model with NMHHC staff and examined NMHHC's organizational structure, physician referral patterns, and patient utilization data. The utilization data indicated that NMHHC currently provides care to substantial numbers of patients with total joint replacements (TJR) and congestive heart failure (CHF). A test of the TM/HLHC model with these particular patient groups is particularly interesting because our *theory* suggests that these two groups, both of whom are high volume users of health care, would experience very different home care outcomes.

TJR patients undergo an elective hospitalization for a surgical procedure that requires substantial amounts of post discharge physical therapy. Although both joint replacement procedures are widely acknowledged to be successful, at present we do not know what effect post-discharge care has on functional status and cost outcomes.

When our study began, 36% of THR patients and 39% of TKR patients hospitalized at Northwestern Memorial Hospital received short term rehabilitation hospital care for approximately seven days following discharge at a cost of approximately $1,000.00/day. If a rehab bed was not available, patients were retained in the hospital for an additional one to two days of acute care. The two surgeons who perform the majority of the TJR procedures have worked with NMHHC to develop a protocol for the aftercare of TJR patients in the home. Because of the high cost of inpatient rehabilitation hospital stays (estimated at a minimum to be $775,000 in FY92), the surgeons want to learn whether a TJR home care protocol that provides more intensive therapy in the first weeks after hospital discharge can substitute for and/or reduce rehabilitation hospital days (thereby reducing costs) and simultaneously produce the same or better functional status outcomes.

Although a recently published review article states that, "patients can usually carry out the (TJR) exercise program at home after initial instructions" (Harris and Sledge, 1990), orthopedic surgeons are hesitant about direct discharge to home care because complications can occur. Particularly for the first three months after surgery, total hip patients are at-risk for dislocation of the hip. If the hip dislocates, the patients must be taken by ambulance back to the hospital to be readmitted for reduction of the dislocated hip which may require a general anaesthetic. The use of a hip abduction brace in the hospital and repeated instructions about hip precautions by nurses and therapists in the inpatient setting have been the main way to prevent this complication.

Deep wound infection is another major post-operative complication that can occur in both hip and knee replacement groups, although it generally occurs in less than 2% of cases. Degree of joint flexion is an important outcome for both procedures, and is especially important in knee replacement patients. If patients do not receive the proper amount and type of physical therapy after hospital discharge, they are at-risk of developing a "frozen" joint that could require manipulation under general anaesthesia to break up adhesions. Thus, the provision of skilled nursing care for wounds and the provision of and compliance with a detailed physical therapy regimen are critical components of any aftercare program provided for these patients. The joint development by an orthopedic surgeon and home care staff of a home care TJR protocol that directly addresses these concerns and the implementation of this protocol by a team of hospital-linked home care providers can be expected to allay these concerns.

In contrast to THR, CHF is a life-threatening condition that accounts for more hospital discharges than any other DRG (Kantrowitz, 1988). Most patients who are hospitalized for treatment of CHF have a New York Heart Association Functional Class score of III or IV (Criteria Committee of the New York Heart Association, 1964). Patients with Class III cardiac disease experience marked limitation of physical activity. Although these patients are comfortable at rest, less than ordinary activity causes fatigue, palpitation, dyspnea or anginal pain. Class IV patients cannot carry on any physical activity without discomfort and symptoms may even be present at rest.

A 1985 study of six-month hospital readmission rates among patients 65 years of age and older found that patients with a primary diagnosis of CHF were at higher risk of hospital readmission than patients with cerebrovascular disease or hip fracture (Gooding and Jette, 1985). Patients with CHF who were admitted for a short stay and discharged directly home and those with atrial and ventricular arrhythmias and uncorrected valve defects were at particular risk. According to the authors: . . . "more aggressive home care after discharge, improved coordination efforts with primary care provider, frequent monitoring, or increased use of step-down facilities such as rehabilitation hospitals might substantially reduce readmission for related causes for this cohort" (Gooding and Jette, 1985).

As this brief review indicates, both persons with TJR surgery and persons hospitalized with a primary diagnosis of CHF appear to be appropriate target populations for a skilled home care intervention.

Both patient populations are eligible for Medicare reimbursed home health care. It seems reasonable that a skilled, *hospital-linked* home care model *that maximizes physician input into the development of condition-specific protocols* would be most successful for these patient groups. Consistent with our theory, different utilization outcomes are likely for the two groups. Specifically, we hypothesized that the provision of TM/HLHC to patients following TJR would reduce *short term rehabilitation hospital admissions*. In contrast, TM/HLHC is expected to reduce *acute hospital readmission days* for the CHF group. These savings were hypothesized to be accompanied by similar or improved patient functional status outcomes, using condition-specific measures.

As this somewhat lengthy example illustrates, a great deal of planning is needed to design a study that is sufficiently sensitive to detect an impact of services on patient outcomes. Thus, outcome studies usually require substantial investments of time, staff and money. Agencies that wish to initiate outcome assessments can benefit greatly by approaching this activity as a collaborative venture with local area academics who can assist with proposal writing and can provide technical assistance with design, measurement, data handling and data analysis issues.

CONCLUSION

As this chapter demonstrates, evaluations come in all shapes and sizes, vary in terms of scope, intensity and complexity and must be tailored carefully to the question of interest. Home care agencies that use evaluation tools and methods will have the capacity to plan and assess services in a very powerful way. Formative and process evaluations can be incorporated with little trouble into ongoing agency operations, especially if agencies designate a staff person with that responsibility. In partnership with academics, considerably more complex outcome evaluations can also be undertaken quite successfully. But why should agencies bother? If anything, the recent national debate over health care reform has taught us that business as usual is unaffordable. We need valid and reliable knowledge about consumers' preferences and about how to provide services that accomplish their intended objectives. Providers are going to be called upon in the future by regulators and by payors to demonstrate that they can assess the quality and effectiveness of services they provide and that the services provide good value for the required investment. Thus, agencies that have the capacity to evaluate their services in these ways will have a definite competitive advantage in this new environment.

REFERENCES

Berwick, D.M. (1989). "Continuous improvement as an ideal in health care." *New England Journal of Medicine*, 320:53-56.

Bobnet, N.L., Ilcyn, J., Milanovich, P.S., Ream, M.A., Wright, K. (1993). "Continuous quality improvement: Improving quality in your home care organization." *JONA*, 23:42-48.

Cummings, J., Hughes, S.L., and Weaver, F.M. "A multi-site randomized trial of team managed VA hospital based home care." Funded by the Department of Veterans Affairs, Cooperative Centers for Studies in Health Services (#3), 1992-1997.

Cummings, J., Hughes, S.L., Weaver, F.M., Manheim, L., Conrad, K., Nash, K., Braun, B. and Adelman, J. (1990). "Cost-effectiveness of V.A. hospital-based home care: A randomized clinical trial." *Archives of Internal Medicine*, (150):1274-80.

Gooding, J. and Jette, A.M. (1985). "Hospital readmissions among the elderly." *Journal of the American Geriatrics Society*, 595-601.

Harris, W.H. and Sledge, C.B. (1990). "Total hip and total knee replacement." (First of Two Parts). *New England Journal of Medicine*, 323(11):725-731.

Hedrick, S.C. and Inui, T.S. (1986). "The Effectiveness and cost of home care: An information synthesis." *Health Services Research*, 20:851-879.

Hughes, S.L., Cummings, J., Weaver, F.M., Manheim, L., Braun, B. and Conrad, K. (1992). "A randomized trial of the cost-effectiveness of home health care for the terminally ill." *Health Services Research*, 26(6):801-17.

Hughes, S.L., Cummings, J., Weaver, F.M., Manheim, L., Conrad, K. and Nash, K. (1990). "A randomized trial of VA home care for severely disabled veterans." *Medical Care*, 28(2):135-145.

Hughes, S.L. (1985). "Apples and oranges? A review of demonstrations and evaluations of community-based long term care." *Health Services Research*, 20(4):461-488.

Hughes, S.L., Cordray, D.S., and Spiker, V.A. (1984). "Evaluation of a long term home care program." *Medical Care*, 22(5):460-475.

Kane, R.A. and Kane, R.L. (1981). *Assessing the Elderly*. Toronto: Lexington Books.

Kantrowitz, A. (1988). "State of the art circulatory support." *Transactions–American Society Artificial Internal Organs*, Vol. 34:445-449.

Kemper, P.R., Applebaum, R., and Harrigan, M. (1988a). "Community care demonstrations: What have we learned?" *Health Care Financing Review*, 8:87-100.

Kemper, P.R., Brown, R.S., Carcagno, G.J., Applebaum, R.A., Christianson, J.B., Corson, W., Dunstan, S.M., Grannemann, T., Harrigan, M., Holden, N., Phillips, B.R., Schore, J., Thornton, C., Wooldridge, J., and Skidmore, F. (1988b). "The evaluation of the National Long-Term Care Demonstration." *Health Services Research*, (special issue) 23.

Leimnetzer, M.J., Ryan, D.A., and Niemann, V.G. (1993). The Hospital-Visiting Nurse Association partnership: A continuous quality improvement program. *JONA*, 23:20-23.

Rust, M.E. (1992). "Home care revival." *American Medical News*, July:23-26.

Ware, J.E. and Sherbourne, C.D. (1992). "The MOS 36-item short-form health survey." *Medical Care*, 30(6):473-481.

Weissert, W.G., Cready, C.M., and Pawelak, J. (1988). "The past and future of home and community-based long-term care." *The Milbank Quarterly*, 66: 309-389.

Chapter 7

Marketing Techniques
for Home Care Programs

Lenard W. Kaye, DSW

INTRODUCTION

The continuing upswing in the number of community programs that provide in-home interventions for the functionally-impaired elderly is being accompanied by a major transformation in the way these agencies carry out their daily administrative responsibilities. Already, many home health care agencies and other health and social service agencies are included among those organizational entities which are embracing an aggressive marketing mentality. In fact, a select group of home health care agencies can be counted among those human service programs which direct considerable resources to the planning, implementation, and promotion of the services they offer. Situated on the leading edge of the marketing function, these home care agencies have already established rather sophisticated approaches to carrying out marketing-related activities. Other agencies, however, are just now coming to realize the importance of services marketing for their long-term organizational survival. Still others are denying altogether the marketing imperative.

This chapter will speak to the importance of home health care

[Haworth co-indexing entry note]: "Marketing Techniques for Home Care Programs." Kaye, Lenard W. Co-published simultaneously in *Journal of Gerontological Social Work* (The Haworth Press, Inc.) Vol. 24, No. 3/4, 1995, pp. 133-156; and: *New Developments in Home Care Services for the Elderly: Innovations in Policy, Program, and Practice* (ed: Lenard W. Kaye) The Haworth Press, Inc., 1995, pp. 133-156. Single or multiple copies of this article are available from The Haworth Document Delivery Service [1-800-342-9678, 9:00 a.m. - 5:00 p.m. (EST)].

© 1995 by The Haworth Press, Inc. All rights reserved. *133*

administrators thinking strategically about their organization's activities and embracing early on a marketing perspective. Marketing in home health care is defined as an ongoing organizational and managerial system designed to plan, promote, and distribute in-home services to populations in need. It will be argued that a thoughtful marketing program better insures that the home health care agency will be able to: compete successfully for consumers; protect themselves against the unexpected loss of public and private revenue; continually generate evidence of demand for service; develop new services and modify old ones in a timely fashion; and insure the building and maintenance of patient enrollment for the agency's long-term financial stability. As an organized strategy for optimizing organizational growth, home health care marketing encourages an agency to arrive at an understanding of: the preferred role it should assume in the field of in-home care; the optimal way in which to utilize available resources to satisfy the needs and demands of consumers; an understanding of the workings of the home health care marketplace; and the requisite strategies for better assuring the success of the organization. It is maintained that a marketing philosophy assists home health care administrators in identifying and satisfying constituent needs at the same time that they preserve the integrity of their organizations. When done properly, better marketing insures that an agency's services will be used. By assuring better service utilization, a marketing perspective is likely to promote the diversification of agency sources of revenue thus increasing the organization's potential for growth and future financial security. It is posited that marketing initiatives are more likely to fail when agencies overlook the need to engage in preliminary planning and research; when they fail to target their efforts accurately; when they lack the necessary financial resources, experience and expertise required to market in the first place; and when they carry unrealistic expectations of the likely consequences of the marketing effort.

Considerable data for this chapter will be drawn generally from two studies of health and social service agency experience, and home health care agency experience in particular; carried out at Bryn Mawr College Graduate School of Social Work and Social Research and supported by the Andrus Foundation of the American

Association of Retired Persons (Kaye and Davitt, 1994; Kaye and Reisman, 1991).

A nontraditional stance will be adopted in discussing the marketing function in home health care. An eclectic approach to marketing is put forward which advocates for broad-based involvement of direct service field staff and service recipients, themselves, in marketing activities. Marketing as an elite function, restricted to the purview of the organizational executive, is rejected outright. Rather, the idea of participatory marketing is developed and deemed particularly appropriate for home care given the significance and centrality of field staff in the service intervention process. Such a perspective speaks to the importance of social workers, nurses, home health aides, other home care agency staff, as well as service recipients performing pivotal functions as part of the marketing enterprise.

For the purposes of this discussion, marketing is characterized as the process by which a home health care agency engages in one or more of the following activities: (1) collecting information about the internal and external environment of the organization; (2) planning ways in which the agency will reach the consumer; (3) developing new services based on consumer need; (4) advertising the service; (5) engaging in public relations; (6) soliciting funds; and (7) recruiting and enrolling clients. Marketing is seen as an organized strategy for optimizing growth by primarily focusing on consumer needs rather than on an available service or product and increasing revenue through consumer satisfaction rather than service volume alone. Put differently, marketing as conceptualized here, aims to embrace a client-oriented focus that, in turn, presses the organization to identify and satisfy client needs in order to survive and prosper. Of course, maintaining adequate consumer enrollment in the agency's repertoire of programs is going to be the ultimate measure of survivability. Given the limitations of space, the emphasis in this chapter will be on a subset of stages comprising the marketing process.

This chapter begins with a summary of major trends serving to escalate in importance the home care marketing function in health and social service programs. The discussion proceeds to an explication of the major benefits derived from program marketing, including its advantages for the home care manager. The reasons why many marketing programs fail are considered, as are the central components of a good home care marketing program including specific strategies for success and the most effective types of home care promotional tools. Major tasks in terms of arriving at a more sophisticated understanding of the uniqueness of individual home health care agency service packages are identified for the reader. Finally, the idea of participatory marketing is further developed. Implications of a marketing mentality in home health care for agency administration, staffing, and direct service delivery are considered throughout the chapter as are issues of practice ethics and client diversity.

THE GROWING IMPORTANCE
OF HOME HEALTH CARE MARKETING

Since the early 1980s, interest in marketing services, as opposed to products, has gained momentum. Early in this evolutionary process, Uhl and Upah (1983) attributed this upsurge in attention to three factors: (1) acknowledgement by marketing professionals that service marketing has unique characteristics; (2) changes in regulations which allow professions previously banned from marketing their services to do so (e.g., health and mental health professionals); and (3) an increase in service expenditures by consumers when compared to product expenditures. Growing numbers, increased longevity, and the improved financial resources of older adults have further reinforced a welcoming environment for traditionally overlooked possibilities in the marketing of services and products to elders in particular (Balazs, Schewe, and Spotts, 1989; Dychtwald and Flower, 1989; Harris, 1988; Lumpkin, Caballero, and Chonko, 1989; Mertz and Stephens, 1990). In addition to the demographic, regulatory, and economic forces driving a marketing mentality in the human services, are those factors generally associated with health and social service programming, including dwindling funds, increased competition, and calls for accountability (Segal, 1991).

Fierce competition appears to be a factor of particular importance in the case of the upsurge in marketing activities within the home health care industry (Sweeney and Wolf, 1989). In the midst of calls to create alternatives to institutionalized care of the elderly and disabled, the increased likelihood of at least partial in-home coverage through private long-term care insurance policies, and the establishment of Medicare's Prospective Payment System, the number of organizations engaged in the delivery of home health care services has grown at a frenetic pace. Hospitals and both regional and national health service corporations are now firmly established players in the home health care arena (Meany-Handy, 1986).

At the same time that older adults may be increasingly apt to be treated at home, they are also likely to have greater choice among a wider range of service alternatives to institutional care. Thus, home care agencies can expect to be competing with health-related facilities, continuing care retirement communities, congregate housing, and related service-enriched residences as well as other community-based interventions such as adult day care, respite, and senior center services. Marketing and planning have been identified as two of the necessary managerial responses to the stresses placed on health care organizations such as home care agencies by the current turbulent service delivery environment (Lee, 1990).

Community service organizations are dealing with an increasingly enlightened elderly consumer population. Elders are more sophisticated and informed and are expressing heightened expectations in terms of the range and quality of service options they wish to have available to them in the community. These same elders express greater increments of self-confidence and control over their lives at the same time that they perceive themselves as younger in age and outlook (Schiffman and Sherman, 1991). Home care agencies are also more likely to be dealing with representatives of older adults who are acting as advocates for their clients. The advent of private geriatric care managers and their nonprofit and public service agency counterparts has resulted in increasing numbers of older persons having rather sophisticated professionals representing and helping them maneuver the service system. Such advocates are likely to have expertise in critically assessing the relative desirability of one home care service versus another. Agencies must therefore be able to market themselves effectively to both well-informed older adults and their professional representatives.

Greater differentiation among home health and home care agencies (e.g., some offer a wide range of high-tech interventions while others focus on low-end services) is also fueling the marketing imperative. Home care is no longer a commodity item. Rather, it is increasingly a specialty service or product which will need to be precisely described and explained to potential consumers in order that the full range of categories of home health care be understood and informed decisions be made ultimately by users.

Finally, the increased use of marketing, particularly professional marketing in the health and human services, is likely not so much to give the agency a competitive advantage as it is to insure the maintenance of a positive image among potential consumers. Indeed, the absence of marketing is bound to be perceived by some consumers as a deficiency in a home care agency's overall operational stance.

THE CENTRAL COMPONENTS OF A GOOD HOME CARE MARKETING PROGRAM

Comprehensive home care marketing encompasses a series of seven discrete components (Kaye, 1992).

Market Research. This phase entails the collection of information about the internal and external environments of the home health care agency. Issues of concern in the external environment include: identifying the level of need for service in a given community; assessing existing in-home services in the community; tracking health and functional impairment trends among potential service beneficiaries; assessing available reimbursement sources; assessing the level of risk in undertaking the offering of a particular service; and profiling the characteristics of the agency's target population(s). Internal agency issues to be considered include assessments of the adequacy of the agency's physical plant, equipment, available capital, staff, information and referral networks, boards and advisory groups, and systems of information management.

Market research is essential particularly when an agency is considering the offering of a new home health care service or the expansion of an existing service. When carried out properly, such an analysis will enable the program planner to determine whether a project under consideration is feasible and likely to be viable if undertaken. Taking the time to carry out preliminary market research, while not without its short-term costs, can, in the long-term, save the home care program planner substantially more time and money.

Marketing Planning and Strategy Development. This phase of marketing provides a general programmatic framework for identifying, collecting, and capturing selected segments of the home care marketplace. For example, it is at this point that a decision might be made to expand the agency's programs to include the provision of hospice care or shopping and attendant services because market research indicated a significant need in a given community. This phase ultimately entails full commitment to the development of a new service (or modification of an existing one). The planner is mindful of taking full advantage of existing opportunities and gaps in the marketplace. The operational details of the program are formulated including philosophy, goals and objectives, service parameters, and resources required. In addition, the agency will want to arrive at decisions concerning what the current predominant "business" of the organization is as well as what is planned as the predominant "business" of the future (Newton and Henry, 1992).

Advertising. This phase differs from public relations in that its focus is on paid communications about the new service offering aimed at influencing the home care market in a given community. Decisions are made concerning the use of broadcast versus print media and mass versus personalized, face-to-face approaches to informing potential consumers of agency services. Advertising efforts may focus on one or more of several goals: attracting more consumers of service; increasing the visibility of the agency in the community; attracting qualified staff; expanding the revenue base; or strengthening the image or perception of the agency held by the public.

Public Relations. This phase focuses primarily on free publicity meant to promote goodwill within the community toward agency services and to insure a clear and positive view of the agency's mission by the larger public. Public relations efforts are realized by way of staff representation on community boards, advisory committees of other agencies, and interagency councils. Staff involvement in community activities that may not be directly related to home care service delivery is also useful so as to nurture a wide range of potentially fruitful contacts and supporters. Staff involvement in community activities is likely to result in identifying and influencing opinion leaders in a given community. Opinion leaders who are not associated directly with a particular home health care agency and who come to realize the benefits of a particular agency's services can become highly influential spokespersons on behalf of a given organization (Williams and Williams, 1988).

Resource Procurement. This phase involves the active solicitation of funds for the agency and the identification of likely sources of reimbursement for services provided. Home care marketing strategy during this stage often includes investigations into the availability of both public and private funds supportive of particular home care program interventions. Funding sources that are likely to be investigated include Medicare, Medicaid, long-term care insurance programs, Medigap programs, and special projects supported through private foundations.

Consumer Relations. This phase of marketing is geared to the home care agency identifying an individual who will act as an intermediary or liaison between the agency and both actual and potential consumers (elderly clients and their relatives). Such an individual has the charge of promoting ongoing positive relations and agency image in the service community.

Sales. The marketing process is completed or closed when clients are enrolled successfully in the home care program.

Agency performance of the previously described phases of home care marketing is driven by answers to the following pivotal marketing questions:

a. What business is the home care agency in?
b. Who are the agency's patients and what kinds of needs do they have?
c. What are the major strengths and weaknesses of the agency's home care program?
d. Who are the agency's major competitors?
e. Which potential client groups in the community offer the best opportunities for the home care agency?
f. What strategies should be developed to maintain an effective and efficient home care service?
g. How can the agency keep abreast of changes in need among the home care consumers it aims to serve?

SPECIAL CHALLENGES FOR THE HOME CARE AGENCY

The dynamic nature of the home health care marketplace and the changing profile of the home care consumer make the following tasks both challenging and essential.

Identifying the Target Population. This activity should be an ongoing one. The demographics of an agency's target population will likely change over time. For financial reasons, certain consumer populations may yield greater return for an agency than others. This happened in the case of nursing homes with the advent of diagnostic related groups (DRGs). Nursing homes preferred certain classifications of patients with diagnoses that yielded the highest reimbursement rates and therefore the highest margins for the organization. Home care agencies, at varying points in time, may also be pressed to identify preferred users of their services for financial reasons.

The changing nature of the configuration of services offered by a home health care organization may also serve to alter the profile of the target population served. For example, the fact that more agencies are likely to offer infusion therapies in the future can alter the characteristics of clients served. Also, new competitors may enter the home care arena while others go out of business. Each time this happens the characteristics of the target population can potentially change. Finally, newly secured funding for special programming other than standard reimbursement can also serve to alter program beneficiary profiles. Timely identification of changes in an agency's consumer profile will insure that publicity and advertising materials can be altered accordingly and thus remain accurate in terms of whom it appeals to.

Market Segmentation. Referred to here is the process of dividing a market into distinct groups of buyers that might require separate services and/or marketing programs directed to them (Green, Tull, and Albaum, 1988). Meaningful market segmentation requires that one determine the perceptions, preferences, characteristics, or other aspects of consumer choice that might differ across buyer groups for particular products or services. The segmentation of markets should contribute to more accurate market targeting by the home care agency. It is essential that the market segmentation process include consideration of all types of consumer diversity including, but not necessarily limited to:

a. race, ethnicity, and religion;
b. gender;
c. age (young old vs. old-old);
d. socioeconomic status;
e. level of education;
f. infirmity/prognosis;
g. intervention preferences (high-tech vs. low-tech, palliative vs. curative, etc.);
h. service decision-maker (self, others, or joint);
i. availability of informal supports.

A thorough market research process should yield comprehensive data on all aspects of buyer group diversity that may impact market segmentation.

Market Positioning. As used here, market positioning deals with the perceptions that buyers hold about alternative marketplace offerings. In the case of home health care, services may be perceived, ordinarily, as custodial by the potential consumer. Should the agency wish to focus on providing high-tech services, its marketing efforts would need to focus on changing the perceptions of consumers to a high-tech definition of care. By doing this successfully, the agency will have differentiated its service both internally and externally (i.e., in relation to other home health care programs in the community). Successful market positioning will result in a home health care agency arriving at a more clear definition of its services which differentiates them from the services available from other home health care agencies in the same geographical area. Service differentiation refers to the agency's capacity to identify components of its program which are unique. By doing this, value is added to what is provided and service utilization is better assured. One home health care agency may differentiate itself from other agencies by identifying with a particular auspice or emphasizing a particular set of services or range of personnel. Other ways of differentiating include focusing on a particular consumer population, catchment area, mode of payment, service coverage schedule, or fee scale.

Identifying the Marketing Team. The home health agency should always maintain an accurate profile of its marketing team. The marketing team is composed of those in-house personnel and/or external consultants who have been designated as contributing to the planning, implementation, and maintenance of the agency's overall marketing strategy. A fully staffed marketing team includes agency players who have expertise in:

a. Providing legal counsel at the point of program start-up.
b. Providing financial management.
c. Providing program management.
d. Promoting program awareness/developing communications tools.
e. Conducting marketing research, gathering information, and performing needs assessments.
f. Generating referrals and enrolling patients.

Agencies will want to conduct periodic audits of the marketing team. Objectives of such an audit include the identification of any missing players, making determinations as to whether skills are duplicated unnecessarily among team members, and conducting assessments of the adequacy of expertise and performance records of individuals comprising the team.

Identifying Competitors. Home care agencies should conduct regular surveys of the competition (i.e., those agencies that are providing similar or substitute services in the same geographic area). It is important to remember that competitors are not only current equivalents in terms of service provision but also potential entrants into the home health marketplace as well as possible programmatic substitutes for an agency's services (e.g., nursing homes, health-related facilities, continuing care retirement communities, congregate housing). There may also be home health agencies which are equivalent in terms of service provision but not true competitors in that they operate under a very different fee scale (e.g., one agency could be subsidized or accept third party reimbursement whereas another agency is completely private pay) or use different financial means tests or applications criteria in determining eligibility for care.

Identifying Sources of Referral. Consumers of home health care services are referred by hospital discharge planners, senior center personnel, information and referral workers, private physicians, caregiver support group leaders, private geriatric care practitioners, Area Agency on Aging staff, relatives, friends, and others. The actual identities of these referral sources for home care agency services are constantly changing. Community agencies come and go, the staff occupying particular positions in those agencies are in flux, and the specific roles and responsibilities of staff within a given organization are subject to change. As a result, referral source directories should be updated regularly. Furthermore, home health care agency staff should recognize the value of establishing and maintaining positive and close professional relationships with community agency referral personnel at the same time that work is undertaken to establish and maintain formal procedures for facilitating reciprocal referrals. Positive relations can prove critical to insuring a continuing flow of appropriate referrals.

FOCUSING HOME CARE MARKETING ON SPECIALIZED TARGETS

As discussed above, one benchmark of sensitive marketing is the identification of particular segments or groups within the consumer population that might use particular home health services. These become the agency's target audiences or key markets. Targeting and segmentation enables the identification of distinct and meaningful subsets of clients. Such activities are performed, based on the assumption that client subsets might require separate marketing efforts in order to be reached successfully.

In the case of home health care, it is likely that the organization will have both primary and secondary markets. Home health services may be used in large part by functionally impaired older adults, the agency's primary market. However, the relatives of such persons are likely also to be using home health care services to help reduce caregiving demands on their own time. Caregiving relatives and others comprising the older person's informal caregiving network might, therefore, be considered a secondary market for the agency. Home health care's primary market, the elders themselves, should not be considered a homogeneous consumer group. Subgroups of older people can be expected to have different market and purchase behaviors. Schewe (1984) and Lazer (1985) maintain that the behavior and attitudes of elders are influenced by their relative levels of physical and mental health. their economic status, and their level of independence.

The previous discussion suggests that the capacity of organizations to segment and target the home health market is likely to serve as an excellent barometer of the relative quality of their marketing efforts. Unfortunately, the majority of home health and other health and human service organizations have tended not to feel that marketing strategies need to differ in terms of the age groups served (Kaye, in press). Nor have agencies tended to undertake specialized approaches to marketing services to particular cohorts of older adults even when they have displayed diversity in terms of gender, minority status, physical or mental health, age, or financial status. This lack of differentiation in the marketing message for subgroups of elder consumers highlights one aspect of human services marketing still situated in an early stage of evolutionary sophistication.

On the other hand, agencies have succeeded in differentiating more clearly when targeting markets other than older persons. While elders are likely to represent the primary, albeit undifferentiated target, community referral agencies, relatives of older adults, and the general public are common secondary targets of marketing efforts. Relatively less attention is directed at friends and neighbors of the elderly, but they too can be the recipients of such agencies' outreach efforts. Health services agencies such as home health care programs are likely, in particular, to market more frequently to relatives of elders as compared to social service organizations (Kaye, in press).

PROMOTIONAL STRATEGIES THAT WORK BEST

Executive directors of home health care agencies and other health and human service organizations report that there are several marketing strategies which they have found to be effective (Kaye and Reisman, 1991; Kaye, 1994). The three most successful methods incorporate face-to-face contact with older persons, their significant others, or their professional representatives and advocates.

They are in-person outreach, group presentations or speeches before community groups and other organizations, and the administration of focus groups with potential consumers of services. Of somewhat lesser value, but useful nevertheless, are printed brochures or program flyers and announcements and direct consumer mailings. In fact, a carefully constructed information brochure or flyer continues to represent an important tool in the hands of the provider of home health care services. Still other organizations have gone the route of using less personal print, radio, and television media, although these strategies are recognized generally to be less precise and effective in reaching highly specialized target audiences.

Because communities differ significantly in their response to particular forms of outreach, a multiplicity of approaches to distributing publicity about an agency's services is strongly recommended. What works for one target population may not work for another.

If an agency does choose to market to their target population by way of a media outlet (newspapers, radio, TV stations, etc.) they should maintain an up-to-date media file (Rose, 1994). Such a file should contain information about the media outlets that best reach the marketing campaign's target audience including: the names, addresses and main telephone number of each outlet; the names, titles, and direct telephone lines of each outlet's decision makers; and summaries of each media outlet's geographical coverage area and its audience.

Regardless of the marketing strategy used for transmitting information about an agency to the larger public, the home care agency will need to make a series of decisions about the manner in which they wish to communicate their message. Can the agency rely on in-house skills in designing advertising and promotional copy or should it turn to a professional ad agency? Is a hard or soft sell more desirable? Should the message be brief and simple or more in-depth and detailed? Is co-marketing with other agencies and/or businesses desirable? These decisions are considered in further detail to follow.

Collaborative Marketing Ventures

Increasingly common are formal collaborative marketing efforts carried out between two or more health and human services organizations. Collaborative ventures in marketing are being fueled in part by a state of resource scarcity in many health service organizations. Multihospital systems and alliances are already commonplace (Coddington and Moore, 1987). It is not uncommon for home health care programs to co-market with local community hospitals, medical centers, neighborhood wellness programs, and other health care organizations. Agencies also commonly collaborate in community education forums, long-term care consortia, joint fund-raisers, and health and service fairs as well as joint meetings convened expressly to share ideas about marketing to consumers. On a more limited basis, joint promotion efforts can occur among two or more service programs or departments within the same agency.

Some agencies have gone a step further and initiated cooperative arrangements with corporations and community businesses in which the latter have underwritten the costs associated with producing annual reports, agency newsletters, service directories, health screening projects, health care education and wellness promotion pamphlets, and other marketing materials and programs. A large corporation or bank may be willing to participate in a matching funds program with a local agency. Joint ventures in marketing have also been undertaken between home health agencies, durable medical equipment companies, and hospitals (businesses often find collaborations with health care providers to be a good strategy for promoting positive relations with the community). Participation by business leaders on home health agency boards of directors and advisory committees represents a commonly utilized mechanism in which to initiate cooperative ventures and/or better utilize the marketing expertise of business professionals. Of course, the home care agency will need to determine whether they wish to become associated with particular sectors and entities within the business community. Such partnerships, should, however, not be dismissed out of hand. Mutual gains can be realized whereby corporate approaches to marketing and public relations enhance the efficiency and effectiveness of the human service agency, just as direct experience can sensitize the corporate sector to the role played by human service agencies in the lives of corporate employees and their families (Schnall, 1989).

Still other agencies have sought celebrity endorsements and used these in their marketing program. Depending on the scope and breadth of agency outreach, such endorsements may be sought from nationally known individuals or widely recognized and respected individuals residing in particular communities. The concept of celebrity is defined broadly here to encompass well-known, long-term residents of a community including physicians, expert authorities, community and business leaders, and respected older adults.

Consumer Views of the Marketing Function

There appears to be considerable consensus across gender, ethnic, socioeconomic, and racial cohorts of older adults as to what approaches by agencies to marketing services are likely to be received most positively. Word-of-mouth appears clearly to be the best method of advertising health and social services to the aged (Kaye and Reisman, 1991; Kaye and Reisman, 1993; Sherman and Forman, 1990). That is, older consumers prefer to use services which are recommended to them personally by people they know and trust, such as relatives and friends. Furthermore, service recommendations from one's personal physician and other professionals in the human services are regarded highly. It is worth noting, however, that the Kaye and Reisman research reflected clear distinctions regarding referral sources between white and African American elders. Whites were found to depend primarily on personal sources of referral (relatives and friends) whereas African Americans relied more heavily on professional referrals. These differences serve to further highlight the importance of variations in specific target populations being taken into account when the home health agency develops its marketing strategy. In any case, consumer preference for personal methods of communicating marketing information through the social and professional networks of a community reinforces earlier agency prescriptions regarding the effectiveness of face-to-face methods of marketing the service message. On the other hand, services which are publicized through commercial and/or broadcast advertising (e.g., telephone "Yellow Pages," television commercials, public billboards) are generally not trusted because they are perceived to have a profit motive driving them. Older adults tend to feel that such advertising is misleading and not particularly informative. Of all forms of marketing, telephone solicitation is perceived most negatively because it represents an uninvited invasion of one's personal space, the home.

Older adults can be expected to be particularly skeptical of the marketing message put forward by proprietary or for-profit agencies. Indeed, elders are capable of making the distinction between advertising carried out for the purposes of "selling" and that which is largely informational. Marketing with a "selling" motive is likely to create feelings of distrust as it may aim to influence persons to purchase or use an unnecessary product or service. Informational marketing is much more likely to be received positively, than more vague, emotional, and abstract appeals that attempt to entertain or unduly influence the potential consumer. Research on the media habits of older people bears this out (Burnett, 1991). For instance, materials which provide advice on how to deal with a particular problem or announce the existence of a new service in the community are more likely to be categorized as educational.

It is important to note that the elder's actual decision to use or not use a service is likely to be driven by the attributes of a described service and more precisely an immediate need for help. In other words, older adults oftentimes do not "shop around" for services in advance of a particular need. This highlights the importance of agency marketing materials making an immediate positive impression if they are to prove successful in drawing a potential consumer to the service. Such materials need to succeed quickly in establishing the trustworthiness of the program and its staff (Quinn and Crabtree, 1987). Because few elders may seek additional information from a service after being exposed to the initial marketing message, it becomes critical that the initial message contains all essential information rather than encouraging them to request further materials.

The Anatomy of Good Promotional Materials

It cannot be overstated that marketing presentation and method have a major influence on how older people perceive service quality. If the marketing medium used by a particular agency does not depict quality in form, the service associated with that medium will inherit the perceived quality or lack thereof.

The quality of the marketing medium is likely to be maximized if home health agencies attend to a series of practical concerns. First, these agencies should take seriously the preferences of their actual and potential consumers. Elders have definite opinions about the manner in which services should be marketed (Kaye, 1995). Specifically, it is recommended that service providers avoid the more commercial media when transmitting information about the programs available to the consumer. Useful program information that assists the older person or his/her relatives or representatives in the decision-making process should be emphasized.

The marketing message when put in print should emphasize the use of high quality, well-contrasting print and paper. Cluttered text and small print should be avoided. On the other hand, visuals and pictures are important aids in promoting recall. While it should be demonstrated and proven to the prospective consumer that the agency in question has certain identifiable advantages, the message should be kept simple (Shewe, 1990; Winston, 1985). Simplicity in communication should be considered paramount given the increasing glut and complexity of information to be found in the elder consumer marketplace. Information provided must be meaningful—that is, it should be accurate, specific, readily comprehensible, relevant, comparative, up-to-date, and available when needed (Mayer and Brady, 1994). Key information including the name of the service and agency, an identified person to contact, and the address and telephone number of the organization in question should be embedded prominently in marketing materials. The overall appearance of the advertisement should be visually pleasing to the eye.

Incorporating authoritative professional endorsements of particular services is encouraged. In addition, elders indicate that they wish the images of older adults in marketing materials to reflect physical and mental vitality but not to the point of distorting the image of the aging experience or the older person. This wish for active images of older persons is to be encouraged even when the services being marketed are specifically geared for functionally impaired elders as in the case of home health care. Portrayals of intergenerational relations are also desirable. All such efforts should aim to minimize stigma for the consumer. Home health care marketers who are sensitive to the positive portrayal of role changes that occur in the later years will be more effective (Schewe and Balazs, 1992) as will those who are sensitive to strategies which reflect an elder's tendency to "think young" (Stephens, 1991).

PARTICIPATORY MARKETING IN HOME HEALTH CARE

Business purists may consider marketing to be primarily a central administrative function with responsibility for its successful performance residing in the offices of home care executive directors or their administrative designees. Indeed, research has confirmed that for the majority of home health care and other health and human service organizations, the planning and implementation of the marketing function resides in the hands of the chief executive. This was the case for 62% of the 274 agencies surveyed by Kaye and Reisman (1991). The second most likely individual bearing responsibility was the individual elder program or project director in larger scale agencies. Less common individuals assigned marketing responsibility were public relations officers, specialized marketing staff, assistant/associate directors, and outside consultants.

Marketing thus appears to be a function assigned to agency elites. Such a perspective is further reinforced by data from the Kaye and Reisman research which confirm that more than half of the organizations surveyed in their analysis (52%) provided "minimal" or "no" opportunities at all for elder contributions to an agency's marketing efforts. Nor was there substantial evidence to suggest that professional and paraprofessional agency staff assumed significant roles in the planning and implementation of marketing agency services.

A participatory marketing stance, on the other hand, speaks to making genuine and widespread use of the range of human resources, both staff and client, that are intrinsic to home health care programming. A participatory marketing mentality values the knowledge and contributions that can be made by individuals providing services in consumers' homes and by individuals consuming those services. It encourages both staff and client to think creatively about marketing and to contribute to the marketing plan in ways which tap their individual capacities.

Using Staff Effectively

A wide variety of staff can and should contribute to an agency's marketing program including: nurses; social workers; occupational, speech, and physical therapists; and home health aides. Their experience on the front lines of service provision provides them with an extremely well-informed perspective on marketing (Kaye, 1992). Such staff have direct access to clients and are, therefore, the most likely recipients of consumer feedback. Such information is extremely valuable as it represents data essential in identifying the changing characteristics of the target population, the identities of potential competitors, and significant gaps in the home care delivery system in a given community.

Both professional and paraprofessional field staff can and should perform an important public relations function. Such individuals will likely have frequent contact with staff affiliated with other organizations, the latter which can serve as important sources for information and referral. Certainly, the reputation that a home health care agency has in the community is influenced heavily by the quality of the working experiences that transpire between that agency's front line staff and the staff employed by other agencies in the community.

Home care staff also are likely to find themselves assuming significant responsibility for maintaining positive consumer relations and serving as liaisons between elder consumers and agency administrators. On occasion, this particular role may extend to their resolving disagreements between client and agency due to the need to interpret, critically, agency policy and procedure. Certainly, field staff will be well aware of the demographic characteristics of clients and their informal networks of family, friends, and neighbors. This can put them in an excellent position to recognize potential targets for agency marketing.

Finally, home care field staff, because of their direct role in service provision, may be particularly well-equipped to think creatively about service innovation. While such persons may lack formal expertise in program planning and development, they probably have a better understanding than anyone else of what clients want. The fact is, administrators are necessarily removed from the daily realities of the service experience and the changing expressions of client need. Yet, effective marketing can hinge on access to this kind of information.

Using Clients Effectively

One measure of the sensitivity of an agency's marketing program is the degree to which consumers, themselves, influence the marketing initiative. Research confirms that older adults have well-established opinions as to what kinds of marketing efforts reflect positively or negatively on an agency's services and ultimately influence their service consumption behavior (Kaye and Reisman, 1993). Unfortunately, elders have been involved minimally in the marketing initiatives of agencies providing health and social services to older persons. Kaye and Reisman (1991) asked executive directors to rate the extent to which elders have participated in such activities. Results confirmed that more than half of the responding organizations (52%) provided "minimal" or "no" opportunities at all for elder contributions to an agency's marketing efforts. Only 17% maintained that older adults participated "very much" in marketing activities.

When older adults have engaged in an agency's marketing program, benefits seemingly accrue to all parties involved. Ways in which elders have participated in the development of agency strategies for marketing services to older persons can range from contributing ideas through focus groups, needs assessments, and patient satisfaction surveys to their involvement as members of agency boards and advisory committees to direct participation by means of the distribution of brochures in local communities, participation in agency phone-a-thons, and other fund-raisers, and member recruitment through informal networking and word-of-mouth (Kaye and Reisman, 1993).

In similar fashion, volunteer assistance can serve as a useful vehicle through which elders give of themselves to the marketing effort. Elder volunteer participation can express itself through such persons posing for publicity photographs to be used in agency brochures as well as writing articles for organizations' newsletters. When their health is not an overwhelming impediment, elders can also participate in community presentations and testimonials which highlight agency services. Agencies can establish special marketing committees comprised of older adults who provide ideas and input around marketing. Older adult membership on an agency's governing or advisory board may also prove to be a common vehicle for assuring elder participation in market planning. There is no reason to assume that simply because elder home care clients are likely to be functionally impaired they are unable to offer legitimate aid to the marketing initiative. The nature of that involvement may simply need to be tailored to coincide with the relative capacity of that client.

CONCLUSIONS

Marketing programs in home health care are now widely endorsed. Less and less negative connotation is attached to those programs that embrace enthusiastically a marketing philosophy. Marketing is quickly becoming a crucial strategy for better insuring survival in today's highly competitive and resource scarce environment regardless whether the home health agency has public, sectarian, nonprofit, or for-profit affiliations. Even so, a number of obstacles need to be overcome if the potential of a marketing perspective is to be realized fully. Perhaps the most significant impediment is the lack of adequate resources such as staff and funding required to mount a meaningful marketing initiative. Other barriers to marketing success include the difficulties inherent in reaching the elderly with the marketing message and overcoming the stigma of service usage felt by some older adults who are resolute in maintaining their autonomy and independence. Additionally, certain personnel in home health and other categories of health and human services may present their own obstacles to successful marketing in the form of negative attitudes concerning the marketing function. Negative attitudes stem in part from prior exposure to insensitive, poorly conceptualized marketing programs by human service programs.

Ultimately, the development of effective marketing initiatives in home health should be seen as impacting positively on consumer enrollment and in turn the future financial security of the organization. When carried out in a thoughtful and well-planned manner, marketing enables the home health care agency to better anticipate and respond to potential changes in the nature and level of competition within the home health services network, changes in government regulation that can impact directly on home care reimbursements, the need to draw qualified employees, and ultimately the likelihood of loss of critical program revenue.

REFERENCES

Balazs, A.L., Schewe, C.D., and Spotts, Jr., H.E. (1989). *An annotated bibliography for marketing to an older population.* Chicago, IL: American Marketing Association.

Burnett, J.J. (1991). "Examining the media habits of the affluent elderly," *Journal of Advertising Research,* October-November, 33-41.

Coddington, D.C. and Moore, K.D. (1987). *Market-driven strategies in health care.* San Francisco, CA: Jossey-Bass Publishers.

Dychtwald, K. and Flower, J. (1989). *Age wave: The challenges and opportunities of an aging America.* Los Angeles, CA: Jeremy P. Tracher, Inc.

Green, P.E., Tull, D.S., and Albaum, G. (1988). *Research for marketing decisions.* Englewood Cliffs, NJ: Prentice Hall.

Harris, H. (1988), "Mature market overview: Marketing the smart house," *International Journal of Technology and Aging,* 1, 67-84.

Kaye, L.W. (in press). "Patterns of targeting and encouraging participation of elder consumers in human services marketing," *Health Marketing Quarterly.*

Kaye, L.W. (1995). "An analysis of promotional materials used by health and social service programs for older adults," *Journal of Nonprofit & Public Sector Marketing,* 3, 17-31.

Kaye, L.W. (1994). "The effectiveness of services marketing: Perceptions of executive directors of gerontological programs," *Administration in Social Work,* 18, 69-85.

Kaye, L.W. (1992). *Home health care.* Newbury Park, CA: Sage Publications, Inc.

Kaye, L.W. and Davitt, J.K. (1994). *High-tech home health care: An analysis of service delivery and consumption.* Bryn Mawr, PA: Bryn Mawr College.

Kaye, L.W. and Reisman, S.I. (1993). "Elder Consumer Preferences of Marketing Strategies in the Human Services," *Health Marketing Quarterly,* 10, 195-210.

Kaye, L.W. and Reisman, S.I. (1991). *A Comparative analysis of marketing services in health and social services for the elderly: Provider and consumer perspectives.* Bryn Mawr, PA: Bryn Mawr College.

Lazer, W. (1986). "Dimensions of the mature market," *Journal of Consumer Marketing,* 3, 23-34.

Lee, J.M. (1990). "Trends in health planning and marketing: A symposium," *Journal of Health and Human Resources Administration,* 12, entire issue.

Lumpkin, J.R., Caballero, M.J., and Chonko, L.B. (1989). *Direct marketing, direct selling, and the mature consumer.* New York, NY: Quorum Books.

Mayer, R.N. and Brady, J.T. (December 1994). *The consumer information research burden: Opportunities and recommendations for lightening the load* (#9413 Public Policy Institute). Washington, DC: American Association of Retired Persons.

Meany-Handy, J. (1986). "Marketing in home health care." In Stuart-Siddall, S. (Ed.), *Home health care nursing: Administrative and clinical perspectives.* Rockville, MD: Aspen Systems Corporation.

Mertz, B. and Stephens, N. (1990). In Schewe, C.D. and Balazs, A.L. (Eds.), *Marketing to an aging population: Selected readings (second edition).* Chicago, IL: American Marketing Association.

Newton, G. and Henry, R.S. (1992). *Marketing adult day programs: Targeting caregivers to reach participants.* Winston-Salem, NC: Bowman Gray School of Medicine of Wake Forest University.

Quinn, T. and Crabtree, J. (June 1987). *How to start a respite service for people with Alzheimer's and their families: A guide for community-based organizations.* New York, NY: The Brookdale Foundation.

Rose, R. (October 1994). "To build clientele, build a media file," *NASW News,* 5.

Segal, U.A. (1991). "Marketing and social welfare: Matched goals and dual constituencies," *Administration in Social Work,* 15, 19-34.

Schewe, C.D. (1990). "Effective communication with our aging population." In Schewe, C.D. and Balazs, A.L. (Eds.), *Marketing to an aging population: Selected readings (second edition).* Chicago, IL: American Marketing Association.

Schewe, C.D. and Balazs, A.L. (1992). "Role transitions in older adults: A marketing opportunity," *Psychology and Marketing,* 9, 85-99.

Sherman, E. and Forman, A. (1990). "The elderly consumer: What do they want and how do they select health care services?" In Schewe, C.D. and Balazs, A.L. (Eds.), *Marketing to an aging population: Selected readings (second edition).* Chicago, IL: American Marketing Association.

Schiffman, L.G. and Sherman, E. (1991). "Value orientations of new-age elderly: The coming of an ageless market," *Journal of Business Research,* 22, 187-194.

Schnall, S.M. (1989). "How big business can help the human services–and vice versa," *Public Welfare,* 47, 6-17.

Stephens, N. (1991). "Cognitive age: A useful concept for advertising," *Journal of Advertising,* XX, 37-48.

Sweeney, R.E. and Wolf, D. (1989). Southern Home Health Care: A case study." In Sweeney, R.E., Berl, R.L., and Winston, W.J. (Eds.), *Cases and select readings in health care marketing.* New York, NY: The Haworth Press, Inc.

Uhl, K. and Upah, G. (1983). "The marketing of services: Why and how is it different?" In Sheth, J. (Ed.), *Research in Marketing.* Greenwich, CT: JAI Press.

Williams, S.D. and Williams, J.R. (1988). *How to market home health care services.* New York, NY: John Wiley & Sons.

Winston, W.J. (1985). "Key points of developing an advertisement for human services." In Winston, W.J. (Ed.), *Marketing strategies for human and social service agencies.* New York, NY: The Haworth Press, Inc.

PART III:
PRACTICE INNOVATION

Chapter 8

Counseling Homebound Clients
and Their Families

Toba Schwaber Kerson, DSW, PhD
Renee W. Michelsen, MSS, LCSW

This chapter has as its focus the means by which social workers and other health care professionals counsel homebound clients and their caregivers. Counseling techniques are presented through a discussion of four case examples which have been chosen to illustrate different social scenarios. The four situations are: (1) a frail elder who wishes to live alone; (2) a terminally ill frail elder whose caregiver is an aged sister; (3) a frail elder with Alzheimer's disease whose family caregiver is her daughter; and (4) a woman with Amyotrophic Lateral Sclerosis whose caregiver is her husband. The case study format is meant to "show the hand" of the counseling professional, to describe exactly how that person intervenes in each scenario. At the end of each case study is a summary of counseling and other interventions. Throughout the chapter, reference is made to the following: counseling the homebound elderly individual, counseling the caregivers, effects of specific illness states, special issues the counselor must address, and always, the necessity for a reasonable availability of concrete services in order for counseling to make any difference in the lives of the homebound elderly.

[Haworth co-indexing entry note]: "Counseling Homebound Clients and Their Families." Kerson, Toba Schwaber, and Renee W. Michelsen. Co-published simultaneously in *Journal of Gerontological Social Work* (The Haworth Press, Inc.) Vol. 24, No. 3/4, 1995, pp. 159-190; and: *New Developments in Home Care Services for the Elderly: Innovations in Policy, Program, and Practice* (ed: Lenard W. Kaye) The Haworth Press, Inc., 1995, pp. 159-190. Single or multiple copies of this article are available from The Haworth Document Delivery Service [1-800-342-9678, 9:00 a.m. - 5:00 p.m. (EST)].

© 1995 by The Haworth Press, Inc. All rights reserved.   *159*

Generally, counseling the homebound elderly and their caregivers is different from counseling other groups for several reasons. First, they have experienced a staggering amount of loss including a significant degree of their own health and physical strength. Perhaps, many peers, a spouse and other friends and family members have died. Often, too, they no longer control many dimensions of life that are considered critical to adult roles in society; they have lost the status acquired in relation to work, earning and other roles in society related to work and earning. Second, the homebound elderly carry a world view and value system often developed in childhood or young adulthood that is not easily understood by the young and middle-aged who provide their care. In addition, they carry a more limited view of the future that is less filled with possibilities and, often, less hopeful. At the same time, they have often attained a distinct kind of wisdom that comes from surviving the exigencies of life. Most of all, no matter how constricted their physical world has become, they maintain a capacity for introspection, psychological and social growth, as well as, an ability to learn from the past (Butler, Lewis and Sunderland, 1991; Hashimi, 1991; Kauffman, 1986; Schlossberg, 1990).

SOURCE OF CASE EXAMPLES

The case examples are drawn from the more than 3,000 cases seen over the last 10 years in an Elder Care Center located in a community hospital in a northeastern suburb. A primary goal of the Center is to help frail elderly people to reside in their own homes as long as they are able to do so in safety. Part of this goal is empowering homebound people to maintain the highest possible level of independence their physical and mental states allow (Kerson, 1989b). Center services include case management, education, a hotline and social work consultation for a county-wide area. Many cases are referred by the local Visiting Nurse Association which provides nursing services and brief social work and other therapy services for which Medicare will pay. When such services are to end, frail elderly individuals are evaluated for case management. (See Chapter 11, "Case Management in Home and Community Care," for an in-depth discussion of case management.)

In terms of case management, the Center provides consultation and management of care for the older individual (Greene and Lewis, 1990; Raiff, 1993; Rothman, 1994). The service begins with an in-home assessment by a social worker who acts as a clinical case manager brokering services and providing counseling to the elder and his or her caregiver (Michelsen, 1989; Morrow-Howell, 1992). This case manager, a specialist in arranging and coordinating community services, helps to identify the needs of the older person and works with the clients to develop a plan of care. Ongoing professional follow-up is provided to ensure that the needs of the elder and family are being met. The case manager is a resource for information and support, providing the elder and family with a single person to call when they have questions or concerns. In regard to social work consultation, the Center provides counseling for caregivers who need help with issues such as coping with caring for an elder, communicating with an elder, coping with Alzheimer's disease, long-range planning, relocating an elder, caring for an elder from a distance, financial and legal concerns, alternative living arrangements, nursing home placement and health insurance. The Telephone Hotline provides information and referral to public and private services and helps callers to identify care options. Finally, the Center provides educational programs on a variety of topics designed for older adults, families, community groups and corporations.

CASE #1:
COUNSELING THE FRAIL ELDER WHO LIVES ALONE

Mrs. Fredericks was an 83 year old white woman, widowed for 21 years, who lived alone in a 200 year old rural farmhouse that had been her home for 50 years. She was referred to the Center by the home care agency nurse who monitored the work of the aides assigned to Mrs. Fredericks. Over the last few years, Mrs. Fredericks had been diagnosed with chronic diverticulitis, osteoporosis, chronic obstructive pulmonary disease, cataracts, a thyroid disorder, high blood pressure, back problems, hearing loss and, most recently, a fractured hip (Roberto, 1992). Approximately eight weeks before the referral, she had been admitted to the hospital for severe abdominal pain due to chronic diverticulitis, and treatment of the condition required an emergency colostomy.

Following her discharge from the hospital, Mrs. Fredericks had lived with her daughter, Adelaide Crawford. Mrs. Crawford and her husband were content to have Mrs. Fredericks with them, but she was determined to return to her own home with the knowledge that she would face many challenges (Hennessy, 1989; Kerson and Zelinka, 1989; Morgan, 1982; Salamon, 1986; Talbott, 1990). Mr. Crawford was Mrs. Crawford's second husband, and although mother-in-law and son-in-law had a good relationship, Mrs. Fredericks felt that her presence placed extra stress on this relatively new marriage.

In terms of activities of daily living, Mrs. Fredericks could dress herself, use the telephone, ambulate with the aid of a walker and use a bedside commode. She required assistance with meal preparation and was unable to bathe herself, shop, keep house, manage her finances or be mobile outside the home. When Mrs. Fredericks was interviewed, she reported no history of mental illness or substance abuse. Before Mrs. Fredericks had become so debilitated, she had been a fine gardener, amateur photographer and a volunteer in a battered women's shelter (Hansson and Carpenter, 1994). When she became too frail to go to the shelter, she made beautiful dolls and afghans for the children who lived there. Mrs. Fredericks' family supported her efforts at independence by visiting, talking to her frequently on the phone, shopping, helping with financial management and transportation. Mrs. Fredericks also continued to receive nursing and home health aide services from the Visiting Nurse Association.

Home Care Counseling

The overarching goal of home care intervention was to help Mrs. Fredericks and her family to negotiate the social service delivery system (Kerson, 1989a). The social worker identified the following services to assist Mrs. Fredericks in remaining independent: an emergency response call system, financial assistance for prescription drugs, home-delivered meals, utility bill assistance, and house cleaning. The family was very eager to have services begin, but Mrs. Fredericks was hesitant (Gatz, Bengtson and Blum, 1990; Norris, Stephens and Kinney, 1990). She was proud of her independence, did not like having a home health aide assist her in bathing and wanted none of the other new services.

The social worker spent the first few visits asking Mrs. Fredericks about her home and admiring her handiwork and photography. Initially, Mrs. Fredericks was very cold towards the social worker seeing the social worker as more aligned with her daughter than herself. Mrs. Fredericks' daughter, Adelaide Crawford, called the social worker and asked that in-home services begin immediately and that arrangements be made for her mother to attend senior citizen club meetings and other social functions. The social worker advised Mrs. Crawford that she heard and understood her concerns, but until Mrs. Fredericks would agree, no services would begin. The social worker emphasized that Mrs. Fredericks had to be the one who was in control, that she had to be the person who accepted or denied services (Rodin and Timko, 1992; Teitelman and Priddy, 1988). Mrs. Fredericks had lost control over many dimensions of her life with the recent exacerbation of her diverticulitis, and it was especially important that she make service decisions. During phone calls and visits to Mrs. Fredericks, the social worker began to understand what independence meant to her. Mrs. Fredericks was embarrassed about her colostomy thinking that it smelled, gurgled and could be seen through her clothing. Consequently, she refused to leave the house. She refused to discuss the colostomy with the social worker preferring to talk to her nurse. She stated that she would not accept "welfare" and did not want any services.

After a few weeks Mrs. Fredericks fell at night and had great difficulty pulling herself to a phone. She was not hurt, but the incident alarmed her and caused her to talk to the social worker. She began to open up slowly and said that sometimes she was frightened at night. The social worker gently reminded Mrs. Fredericks that the purpose of the services was to support her independence not to take it away. Shortly afterwards, Mrs. Fredericks agreed to an emergency response system. She was very happy with the sense of security that it gave her.

One of the most important ways in which the social worker engaged Mrs. Fredericks was through pet therapy (Cox, 1992; Davis, 1987; Meen, 1987). The social worker has a well-trained and friendly dog who, with advanced permission from the clients, sometimes accompanies the social worker on her visits. The social worker had learned previously that Mrs. Fredericks was very fond of dogs, and Mrs. Fredericks was amused to find that the social worker's dog and she had something in common; they were both named Charlotte. Charlotte, the dog, was so successful in helping to lift Mrs. Fredericks' depression that the social worker arranged to have a pet therapy volunteer and her dog visit Mrs. Fredericks once a week.

The next hurdle was home-delivered meals. It was getting more complicated for Mrs. Crawford, who had just returned to work, to bring meals to her mother's house. In fact, Mrs. Crawford often arrived angry and shouted that if her mother had only agreed to live with her, all of this could have been avoided. The social worker helped Mrs. Fredericks agree to a trial period of meals by pointing out that it would reduce her daughter's stress level and, as a consequence, her daughter might be able to relax a little and stop shouting.

Throughout the process of arranging the concrete services the social worker became more aware of how much Mrs. Fredericks needed to be in control. For example, the day's meals were to be delivered at noon. If they had not arrived by five minutes after noon, Mrs. Fredericks would call to cancel them for the day because she wanted her lunch precisely at noon. As Mrs. Fredericks realized that the social worker was not going to try to take control away from her she began to be more expressive and less guarded. In this way, the social worker could help Mrs. Fredericks rehearse the questions that she wanted to ask both the visiting nurse and her physician, especially regarding the colostomy. Importantly, the social worker helped Mrs. Fredericks to leave the house. First, she asked Mrs. Fredericks to show her her perennial garden. Then, they began to take longer walks across the yard, down the street and around the block, always accompanied by Charlotte, the dog, of course. After several weeks, Mrs. Fredericks accepted an invitation for lunch at a friend's house.

Over time, Mrs. Fredericks regained strength, confidence and control. Gradually Mrs. Fredericks accepted the array of services she required to maintain independence. Once services were routinized, she assumed responsibility for managing her own care. She was clear that she could resume case management services at any time and had the telephone number and other information about the Center, home health aide service, emergency response system, home-delivered meals and the pet therapy volunteer beside her telephone. Case management services were terminated after six months.

Summary of the Counselor's Role

This is a situation in which the social worker began where the client was, kept the empowerment of the client as a central focus and helped the family to learn to follow the cadence of the client in terms of decision making (Compton and Galaway, 1994; Woods and Hollis, 1990). The primary client, Mrs. Fredericks, had to be helped by the social worker to take full measure of herself, to face her losses and to evaluate the level of independence she could maintain and what kinds of supports she needed (Hansson, Remonder and Galusha, 1993). The importance of understanding the illness and its particular impact on such intimate relationships is a central theme here. None of Mrs. Fredericks' physical problems affected her ability to decide for herself what she wanted.

Much of the beginning counseling related to helping Mrs. Crawford give Mrs. Fredericks the time to accept the need for service and then, to accept the services. Psychologically, Mrs. Crawford was moving more rapidly than her mother. Since her mother was the primary client, it was important to have services reflect her need and timing and to help Mrs. Crawford to accept this. In time, Mrs. Fredericks surprised her family by regaining much of her strength and independence. For the time being, she could, indeed, be her own case manager.

CASE STUDY #2:
COUNSELING AN ELDER WHO IS TERMINALLY ILL AND HER CAREGIVER

Mrs. Washington was an 82 year old African American woman who was referred to the Center for in-home follow-up and case management following inpatient radiation treatments. She received services for one year. Mrs. Washington had just completed a series of radiation treatments and had declined services from hospice. She was aware of her diagnosis of metastatic breast cancer and her prognosis, but felt that "hospice services concentrated too much on dying." In-home services were to consist of nursing and home health aides provided by the Visiting Nurses Association and social work services provided by the Center.

Mrs. Washington lived alone in her own large, but deteriorating home, in a suburban neighborhood. Many of her neighbors had moved away and she had been estranged from her church for several years. Primary supports consisted of an elderly sister who had come to stay with her temporarily and a granddaughter who had young children and lived in a near-by state. Four other grandchildren were quite dysfunctional and unable to help. The family had converted a dining room into a room for Mrs. Washington, equipped with a hospital bed, wheelchair and commode.

Mrs. Washington was extremely limited in her mobility due to metastasis of the cancer to the bone. She had a history of falling and was not able to transfer from the bed to a chair or commode without assistance. She was dependent or needed assistance in all activities of daily living except eating. She was able to take her own medication and use the phone but was dependent in activities such as shopping, home cleaning, financial management, and meal preparation. Mrs. Washington was also severely visually impaired. Her sister had assumed the caregiving responsibilities but was overwhelmed and not sure how long she could continue. She scored 80% correct on a mini mental status examination and was fully oriented.

Home Care Counseling

Mrs. Washington was assigned to a young male, white social worker (Beckett and Dungee-Anderson, 1989; Yeatts, 1992; York, 1994). They discussed their racial, sex and age differences, and while Mrs. Washington assured the social worker the differences made no difference to her, he remained sensitive (Proctor and Davis, 1994; Smyer, Zarit and Qualls, 1990). Initial home visits were made in order to provide and coordinate concrete services. Mrs.

Washington and her family wanted an easier way to help her to leave the house–they had been carrying her down the stairs. The social worker referred Mrs. Washington to an agency which had received funding to carry out home repairs and improvements. The agency agreed to build a ramp so that Mrs. Washington could more easily leave the house in her wheelchair. Mrs. Washington and her family were more open to social work counseling after this process began. The visiting nurse managed all of the home health needs of the patient and the social worker continued to focus on emotional and social services issues.

The social worker visited Mrs. Washington once or twice each week. As Mrs. Washington's illness progressed, she began to talk more about dying and the fear of dying. She expressed anger about having this fate, although she had outlived many of her friends and relatives. Sometimes she went into denial saying she was not really terminally ill. Most of the time she was sad. She spoke to the social worker more freely as time passed because she did not want to burden her sister who was already on the brink of leaving.

Mrs. Washington's sister and primary caregiver, Victoria Johnson, was 80 years old, lived in another town and had no other responsibilities. Mrs. Johnson confessed to the social worker many times that the level of care needed by her sister, such as changing diapers and moving from bed to chair or wheelchair was physically beyond her. She was overwhelmed, exhausted, and isolated because she and her sister had few visitors. To show her feelings, she banged the pots and slammed cabinet doors as she cleaned the kitchen. The social worker and Mrs. Washington knew how frustrated she was. The social worker tried to befriend her but she did not want to talk. The social worker finally decided that her visits provided a time for Mrs. Johnson to be by herself. To allow herself a way out, she frequently threatened to leave, but she never did.

The social worker encouraged Mrs. Washington to express her feelings and fears of death and validated their legitimacy. He also helped her to identify ways in which she could feel the most alive. The techniques of reminiscence and life review were highly effective with this client (Beaver, 1991; Butler, 1974; Wallace, 1992). These techniques are about the uses people make of their memories and the forms the reminiscences take. Reminiscence is a normal activity in any age but has particular meaning in old age. Life review, in particular, is a process people use to come to terms with the ways in which they have lived their lives. The use of these techniques can be fragmentary or highly structured. In addition, some people are not concerned with reminiscence, and, in fact, deny its importance, believing that there are other ways to cope with old age and/or disability. Reminiscence makes some people sad or angry and others happy. People's use of these techniques is as different as they are.

Discussion of her earlier life and accomplishments helped Mrs. Washington feel less stressed and realize that the sum of her existence was much more than her current situation. The stories she told the social worker about her past also provided insights about her strengths as a mediator and peacemaker in her family (Saleeby, 1994). This also helped the social worker to understand why the client worried constantly that she was causing people trouble and thought that she should never complain about her plight.

At the beginning of each visit, the worker asked Mrs. Washington how she was feeling. Each time, Mrs. Washington responded that she felt like a burden and hated being taken care of. She never complained of pain. She spoke of how she wished she could "do for herself." The social worker helped her to list all of the things that she was able to do currently in order to help her to see that she was not totally dependent. Again, reminiscence therapy was used here to remind her that she had not always been in this compromised state and had accomplished much in her life. It was important for the social worker to understand how Mrs. Washington used reminiscence and the ways in which it related to her present adjustment to the exigencies of life (Coleman, 1986; Merriam, 1989). For example, Mrs. Washington was very proud that she had earned a high school degree by going to night school. Also, the techniques of positive visual imagery and the relaxation response helped her to feel less depressed and anxious (Benson, 1992; Dossey, 1985; Overholser, 1991; Weinberger, 1991). Mrs. Washington stated repeatedly that she wanted to escape her situation, and these techniques helped her to transcend the immediate and find some peace.

The ramp became a joint venture between Mrs. Washington and

the social worker, as Mrs. Washington just wanted to go outside. There were many structural complications and delays in the construction. As the months passed and winter came Mrs. Washington was increasingly bed bound. Her mental abilities were still fully intact, but she was more depressed and felt more and more like a burden. Mrs. Washington told the social worker that on top of everything else, she was bored. It was clear that she lacked stimulation. The social worker discussed anti-depressant medication with her physician, but Mrs. Washington was already on so many medications that he did not want her to take another. Mrs. Washington also reported feeling useless. The social worker suggested having an elder volunteer visit her and read to her if she wished, but she said she did not want new company (Cox and Parsons, 1992). He also suggested that he bring her audiobooks to help her to think about something other than her own situation for a brief time. At first she refused saying that she did not want services for the blind. Through the persistence of the social worker she agreed. He brought a recorded book and tape recorder along for visit and simply left them there for her to try. The books gave her the escape she needed and helped to lift her spirits.

The social worker asked Mrs. Washington whether there was any "unfinished business" with which he could help her. She eventually mentioned that she had stopped going to church but prayed daily on her own and found comfort in prayer. When the social worker suggested calling her minister she adamantly refused. The church topic initiated Mrs. Washington to reminisce about her life history and the events that shaped her. The social worker listened as Mrs. Washington described her strength in times of great adversity. In turn, he pointed out that this strength had also helped her in coping with her illness. They also discussed the importance of church in Mrs. Washington's earlier life.

Towards the end of Mrs. Washington's life she gave the social worker permission to call her minister (Tobin, 1991). The minister visited and in very moving meetings he and Mrs. Washington overcame whatever differences they had in the past. Mrs. Washington's health failed rapidly and she passed away at home.

Summary of the Counselor's Role

The social worker felt that he had helped Mrs. Washington through his consistency, non-judgmental listening, and helping her to put closure on her life. Mrs. Johnson did not want the kind of relationship that the social worker felt was usual for caregivers, and the social worker respected her right to determine the nature of the relationship. Reminiscence therapy was a key to much of the work that Mrs. Washington and the social worker completed. In fact, it was through reminiscence that Mrs. Washington allowed the social worker to contact her minister so that she could rectify her relationship with him and her church. At Mrs. Washington's funeral, the social worker felt sad yet peaceful.

CASE STUDY #3:
COUNSELING ELDER AND CHILD
WHEN THE ELDER HAS ALZHEIMER'S DISEASE

Marjorie Madison was a 77 year old white woman who was referred to the Center by her physician. Mrs. Madison was diagnosed with Alzheimer's Disease and in need of community-based support services (Kerson and Kerson, 1985; Mercer and Robinson, 1989). At the time of the referral, Mrs. Madison had been divorced for many years and resided by herself in a garden apartment. Her only daughter, Jane Broderick, lived nearby, worked full-time as a teacher, managed a household, two school-age children, and a marriage, and was a student in a Master of Education program. It had not been necessary for Mrs. Broderick to be involved in Mrs. Madison's daily life activities until Mrs. Madison began to have memory difficulty and would call her daughter in a confused mental state. In addition, Mrs. Madison's personal hygiene had begun to suffer as had the condition of her apartment.

Comprehensive Office Assessment

Mrs. Madison had a comprehensive assessment by a professional team including physician, nurse and social worker. The assessment included standard of care laboratory tests, magnetic resonance imaging, the Folstein mental status exam, a functional assessment of Activities of Daily Living (ADLs) and Instrumental Activities of Daily Living (IADLs), and an assessment of the family system. As a result of the assessment, the diagnosis of Alzheimer's disease was confirmed. It was determined that Mrs. Madison was in the middle stage of the disease.

Mrs. Broderick was overwhelmed with the level of care that her mother now needed (Jackson, 1993). From Mrs. Broderick's perspective, she and her mother had moved from an aloof, casual relationship to one of total dependence (Dura, Stukenberg and Kiecolt-Glaser, 1991; Gatz, Bengtson and Blum, 1990). Mrs. Broderick sought assistance from the Center on the recommendation of Mrs. Madison's primary physician, and the comprehensive assessment team.

Home Care Counseling

With extensive knowledge gleaned from the comprehensive assessment, the social worker met Mrs. Madison and Mrs. Broderick in Mrs. Madison's home in order to assess Mrs. Madison's living arrangements, her ability to cope in her own home, her relationship with her daughter and, with the goal of arranging and coordinating community services. The home assessment provided many clues to Mrs. Madison's functional and safety status that could not be known in the office setting. The social worker had the task of identifying these clues and interpreting them while respecting Mrs. Madison's privacy. In Mrs. Madison's case, the social worker observed the following. Mrs. Madison was fully ambulatory and not physically incapacitated; yet, she was wearing a soiled nightgown in the afternoon. The day was warm, but the apartment was dark, the curtains were drawn and the windows, closed. The apartment was so humid that mildew grew on the ceiling. Papers and mail were stacked high. The kitchen looked unused, and when Mrs. Madison opened the refrigerator, food emitted a spoiled odor. The bedroom seemed untouched, and the living room couch held blankets and pillow. In this first meeting, the social worker could more precisely define areas of difficulty.

This initial social work interview included an analysis of Mrs.

Madison's functioning. The interview covered questions which would help to assess Mrs. Madison's living conditions, physical health, functional status, mental status including cognitive functioning, history of psychiatric problems and/or substance abuse, community service utilization and financial resources, Mrs. Broderick's and Mrs. Madison's understanding of the diagnosis and prognosis of Alzheimer's disease, and their ability to cope with the diagnosis and Mrs. Madison's care (Mohide et al., 1990).

Mrs. Broderick's sophisticated understanding of Alzheimer's disease greatly frightened her. She could foresee the level of care that her mother would need and was prospectively overwhelmed by the circumstances. Before this meeting, she had not allowed herself to comprehend how deteriorated her mother had become. The home assessment, and listening to Mrs. Madison answer the social worker's questions, helped Mrs. Broderick to see how much help her mother needed. In these situations the older person is the agency's primary client, but the family/caregiver is a very important client as well as a critical member of the caregiving team (Rathbone-McCuan, 1991; Zook, 1992). The social worker found that Mrs. Madison had not previously used any community services. Also her financial resources, at that point, were such that she could pay for services and did not qualify for public assistance.

The social worker reviewed the community programs and services that could immediately provide assistance. Mrs. Madison's level of dementia presented a problem. She did not comprehend her own needs; therefore, she denied needing any assistance. For example, in regard to home-delivered meals, Mrs. Madison made statements such as, "that's a wonderful service, but I prepare three healthy meals for myself daily." This type of reaction is typical for an individual with early to mid-stage Alzheimer's disease. One challenge of working with individuals with Alzheimer's disease is that their ability to reason is obliterated by the disease; so that, intervention strategies must be very different from those used with patients who can rationally make decisions. In this case the social worker maintained Mrs. Madison's dignity by saying that the meals would just be a supplement and good for the days when she felt somewhat "under the weather" (Goldstein, 1983). Mrs. Madison then agreed to try the meals. The social worker observed that Mrs.

Madison was fatigued and distracted. Mrs. Broderick agreed to meet with the social worker separately to discuss required services.

While it was essential for Mrs. Madison to be involved in the care planning process as much as possible, lack of short-term memory caused Mrs. Madison to forget any agreements she made with the social worker in regard to accepting services. Still, depending on the level of Mrs. Madison's dementia, the relationship between Mrs. Madison and the social worker is essential to her trusting the social worker to help her and to cooperating with the social worker and the plan. In the earlier stages of dementia, Mrs. Madison was more able to participate in decision making, but increasingly, decisions had to be made in Mrs. Madison's best interest by a surrogate decision maker, in this case Mrs. Broderick (Abramson, 1988).

Working with Close Relatives

Next, Mrs. Broderick and the social worker met together. In this particular situation, Mrs. Broderick had previously obtained Durable Power of Attorney, which legally allowed her to manage Mrs. Madison's finances and make decisions regarding her care (Bulcroft, Kielkoph, and Tripp, 1991). In situations where families are not so prepared, legal issues present a greater challenge, potentially involving the arduous process of court-appointed guardianship (Iris, 1988; Keith and Wacker, 1994; Soskis and Kerson, 1992). As a way to review their progress and begin the next stage of their work together, the social worker again explained the continuum of available services. Together, the social worker and Mrs. Broderick developed an eco-map to explore available services and supports (Hartman, 1994; Gilgun, 1994). As they developed the care plan in which the social worker explored the level of support the family system could provide for Mrs. Madison, such as morning visits to give medication and managing financial matters, taking Mrs. Madison to her physicians' appointments, or providing transportation to an adult-day-care center; Mrs. Broderick began to weep. Depression and loss remained major themes in her work with the social worker (Walker, Martin and Jones, 1992; Dura, Stukenberg and Kiecolt-Glaser, 1991). She was already doing more than she could manage with her job, husband, small children and other household responsibilities (Brakman, 1994). Although she felt obligated to her mother, mother and daughter had never been close, and Mrs. Broderick cried that this was "too much." In the past, Mrs. Broderick had promised her mother that "she would never place her in a nursing home," but she didn't see how she could handle this (Gubrium, 1991).

The social worker's role now had to be defined in terms of counseling needs and the provision of concrete services. Since in this organization the social worker's role is called case manager, she used her counseling skills to coordinate services for Mrs. Madison, her primary client. However, in order to provide such services, the social worker also had to counsel Mrs. Broderick. If Mrs. Broderick's needs were not met, she may have been unable to do what her mother needed. Indeed, in some cases, the primary caregiver might even have sabotaged the best possible plans if her own needs were not addressed (Pearlman and Crown, 1992; Zarit, 1990). The social worker knew that Mrs. Madison would gain support through the social worker's strengthening the family system. Thus, the social worker discussed individual counseling and caregiver support groups with Mrs. Broderick, who responded that she did not have time for anything that formal and just needed to get these things done (Labrecque, Peak and Toseland, 1992; Toseland, Rossiter, Peak and Smith, 1990).

Through the provision of essential concrete services, the social worker gained the trust of mother and daughter. A complex plan of community services included home-delivered meals, a home health aide for personal care, transportation and adult day care three times a week, and a cleaning service. As a result, the social worker was perceived by the family as a resource. As time progressed the social worker developed a relationship of trust with Mrs. Madison through home visits. Although she was obviously impaired and did not always remember the social worker's name, Mrs. Madison recognized the social worker as safe and an ally. In partnership with Mrs. Broderick, the social worker coordinated services.

Counseling Support for Mrs. Broderick

The social worker became the primary support for Mrs. Broderick who related that her husband was upset by the number of hours she spent caring for her mother (Ganzer and England, 1994; McCallion, Toseland and Diehl, 1994). As Mrs. Madison's disease progressed, Mrs. Broderick became more stressed as did her whole family system. She was more irritable with her children and her family felt neglected. Many more personal calls at work were interfering with her ability to focus. Mr. Broderick was now also checking on his mother-in-law, and Mrs. Broderick now saw her mother and her problems as monopolizing their lives (Tennstedt, McKinlay and Sullivan, 1989).

The social worker helped Mrs. Broderick by using a cognitive, problem-solving approach (Kent, 1990; Lowy, 1985). Part of the work was helping Mrs. Broderick to partialize her problems (Compton and Galaway, 1994). Together they listed all caregiving activities and then determined which were most important for Mrs. Broderick to do herself, which she could delegate to professional providers or other informal resources and which she could eliminate. For example, she recounted that when she shopped for her mother's food, she would place an item in the basket then decide her mother would probably refuse to eat it anyway, or she would decide something was too expensive and put it back, or pick something that was on sale, then think she should not be trying to save money in buying food for her mother. Every food-shopping occasion became one in which to obsess, build resentment and feel paralyzing guilt; so, the social worker arranged for a shopping service to buy and deliver Mrs. Madison's groceries. In addition, Mrs. Broderick expected to maintain the same perfectionistic level of housekeeping and dress for her mother that her mother had had before becoming demented. This added to her stress and meant that she was constantly bickering with her mother's excellent home health aide, Sarah Benson. In addition to being devoted to Mrs. Madison, Mrs. Benson was the only person who could convince Mrs. Madison to shower; however, she did not change Mrs. Madison's nightgown as often as Mrs. Broderick wished. After some discussion with the social worker, Mrs. Broderick developed more realistic expectations. In addition, she decided that while Mrs. Madison appreciated her visits, it was reasonable to come four times a week rather than every day, and it was fine to visit for one hour rather than four hours each time. On the other three days, the aide reminded Mrs. Madison to take the medicine which her daughter had placed in a special pill box container. As a result, the whole situation became less overwhelming for Mrs. Broderick.

When Mrs. Broderick felt more in control, she was able to approach her feelings toward her mother and expressed anger at the mother's ingratitude. She felt that she was giving more than she had ever gotten from her mother, even when she was a little girl. Since her mother had not always supported her in the past, how much did she owe her anyway. She recounted that, except for graduations, her mother had never come to school to see her do anything–even events such as elementary school plays. Her mother never made a fuss about holidays or birthdays and had her shop for herself years before her friends' mothers would even let them buy anything without their express permission. This was not confidence in her daughter, Mrs. Broderick said, but a total lack of caring. For years, Mrs. Broderick harbored hope that, in time, her mother would at least be able to be a friend to her. However, her mother was not supportive of her in her divorce, had stated that her returning to school was a waste of time, and disapproved of her remarriage.

Mrs. Broderick was angry at the disease for placing her in this position and angry at the medical profession for not being able to cure it. She felt her mother was acting this way to get back at her for something. The social worker reviewed the fact that dementia renders the victim incapable of such complex responses. Through a series of discussions Mrs. Broderick was able to better understand her emotions and explore feelings that she had not verbalized before. Mrs. Broderick yearned to create a relationship that never was and wanted recognition that she had never received from her mother (Candib, 1994). Now, she grieved for a relationship that had never been and could never be.

Through their many discussions, the social worker held to the belief that each person had the right to make her own caregiving decisions and that since people's life experiences and responsibilities differed, no societal standard could apply to everyone. Mrs. Broderick agreed to attend a caregivers' support group which, along with telephone supportive counseling from the social worker and bi-weekly meetings at Mrs. Madison's home, allowed her to feel more in control of her emotions. The caregivers' support group, composed of relatives and friends caring for Alzheimer's patients, provided Mrs. Broderick with strength and courage and helped her to alleviate her anxiety and depression (Greene and Monahan, 1989). The group met bi-weekly at a local church in the evening and was convened and led by a professional (Toseland, Rossiter and Labrecque, 1989; Getzel, 1982). The members shared their experiences and the ways in which they had each coped with similar problems at the various stages of the disease. They all discussed the problem of mourning a person who is still alive, and the ongoing hope that it will all be better tomorrow. Through the group and individual counseling, Mrs. Broderick found ways to address her pain; old and new. At that point, she experienced less stress even though her mother continued to deteriorate.

These experiences freed Mrs. Broderick to more seriously consider her mother's moving to a nursing home (Gonyea and Silverstein, 1991). Still hoping that her mother could somehow rise to this occasion, she wanted her mother to tell her she had been a good daughter and that she was right to place her. The "empty chair" technique was used to help Mrs. Broderick express some of her feelings that her mother was no longer capable of understanding (Perls, Hefferline and Goodman, 1951; Polster and Polster, 1974). Mrs. Madison had been receiving Center services for four years. The counseling role was then focused on the guilt Mrs. Broderick had about breaking a promise to her mother. Through the support group and talk with the social worker, Mrs. Broderick came to the realization that when she made the promise she never could have predicted this situation. The social worker helped Mrs. Broderick to explore what her mother had wished to accomplish through this promise. Mrs. Broderick came to the conclusion that her mother wanted to be cared for and protected. In fact, Mrs. Broderick could continue her role as protector and advocate for her mother when her mother lived in a nursing home just as she had while her mother was maintained in her own home.

During the years in which she had received home care, Mrs. Madison had exhausted her financial resources. She was now eligible to apply for Medicaid. The social worker was the primary support person for Mrs. Broderick throughout this long bureaucratic process. Mrs. Broderick continued to attend a support group after the mother was placed and became very helpful to other caregivers.

Summary of the Counselor's Role

The social worker initially focused on the concrete needs of her primary client. Through partnership building, she gained the trust of Mrs. Broderick, her secondary client. In order to counsel both clients, the social worker established a trusting, supportive relationship by providing concrete services. As Mrs. Madison's mental state continued to deteriorate, the social worker's primary counseling responsibility was to her daughter, Mrs. Broderick. Mrs. Broderick initially refused any kind of counseling, but as her mother's condition worsened and she grew closer to the social worker, she worked directly with the social worker on many deep psychological issues and received further social and psychological support from a peer support group. Loss and depression remained themes throughout the work, and Mrs. Broderick was able to resolve much of her anger towards her mother and the guilt she felt at having to place her mother in a nursing home. The psychological and social support Mrs. Broderick received from the social worker in regard to her mother, in fact, empowered her to better manage other dimensions of her life.

CASE #4:
COUNSELING A COUPLE WHEN THE WOMAN HAS AMYOTROPHIC LATERAL SCLEROSIS

Mr. and Mrs. Singer, ages 68 and 65, and married for 45 years, live in a suburban garden apartment complex. Mrs. Singer was referred to the Elder Care Center by a Visiting Nurse Association social worker. She had been hospitalized after fracturing a hip as a result of falling down a flight of stairs at her daughter's home. When she was transferred to a rehabilitation facility for physical therapy, it was noted that Mrs. Singer had marked weakness on one side and muscle twitching. She also reported muscle cramps and a generalized weakness, along with falling, that she had not previously shared with her physician. Extensive testing confirmed a diagnosis of amyotrophic lateral sclerosis (ALS).

Mrs. Singer was followed at home by a VNA nurse, physical therapist and occupational therapist. After several weeks, her condition was considered stable to the point that Medicare would not consider her needing "skilled" nursing care. She had already consumed the limited social work services which Medicare would reimburse, and she was referred to Elder Care for ongoing social work services.

Home Care Counseling

The social worker began her work with a great deal of knowledge about the Singers which had been passed on to Elder Care in the referral process by the VNA social worker. The client had given permission for the information to be shared. Mrs. Singer told the social worker that she had been nervous ever since receiving her diagnosis and found out that the disease was progressive. Using a walker she was walking short distances, she often needed assistance rising from a chair and sometimes required a wheelchair. The VNA therapists had made the apartment handicapped-accessible. Mrs. Singer was able to feed herself, although she often spilled the food and was embarrassed. Mr. Singer assumed most of the IADLs, such as shopping and meal preparation. He was very sad about his wife's diagnosis and prognosis. Mr. Singer was an engineer, now working part-time, and had planned to retire completely in a few months. Prior to receiving Mrs. Singer's diagnosis, the couple had planned a trip to Europe and was thinking of relocating to Arizona. Mrs. Singer was an art teacher, and many of her works were displayed in the apartment.

On her first visit, the social worker spent time admiring Mrs. Singer's art and having Mrs. Singer tell her about individual pieces. She also encouraged Mr. Singer to hire a home health aide to stay with his wife while he was out of the house. Mrs. Singer liked the home health aide but felt increasingly bored with her existence. As a result of discussions with the Singers, the social worker identified the following issues that had to be addressed: the Singers' grief about the illness, its prognosis and the loss of their planned future, and Mrs. Singer's feeling bored and worthless. The Singers welcomed the opportunity to express their feelings.

The social worker first addressed Mrs. Singer's need for stimulation by asking if the couple knew anything about adult day care. Mrs. Singer responded that she didn't want to spend her day with people who were old and confused; she had never really seen an adult day care center and was willing to look at some brochures the social worker promised to send her. When the Singers received the brochures along with a friendly note of encouragement, Mr. Singer called to thank the social worker and asked to speak to her alone at her office.

At that appointment, Mr. Singer was very tearful; he realized how much care his wife would soon need and was afraid he could not manage (Barusch, 1988; Skaff and Pearlin, 1992). He said he was "keeping up a strong front" for his wife so that she could be brave (Rubenstein, 1989). The social worker asked him if he had cried with his wife. He said that he had not, but that he had comforted her on several occasions. The social worker explored the history of the Singers' relationship with Mr. Singer. He thought they had always faced tragedies together, but in this one, he felt alone. The social worker validated Mr. Singer's feelings of loss helping him to enumerate all the losses and potential losses he was experiencing (Brown, 1990; Hooyman and Kiyak, 1988; Simos, 1979). This exercise helped him to increase his understanding of his own feelings. The social worker asked what he thought would happen if he shared his feelings with his wife. He responded that she might be so sad he might not be able to console her. The social worker wondered aloud whether his "strong front" might be creating a distance between Mr. and Mrs. Singer so that neither could express his or her great sadness or anger, and therefore neither could truly comfort the other. Mr. Singer said he did feel a rift between them; they were more formal with each other and "walking on eggs," which was not typical of their relationship. He said he really wanted to reach out to his wife. The social worker gave him the homework assignment of trying to tell his wife how sad and afraid he is. The social worker said Mr. Singer should call her if he needed support or if Mrs. Singer was inconsolable. Mr. Singer was frightened of this direct approach, but he gathered his courage and agreed to try.

Over the next few weeks, Mr. and Mrs. Singer were more able to communicate honestly with each other and, as a result, both were less anxious. Mrs. Singer felt better because she helped her husband contend with his feelings, and Mr. Singer felt less isolated and emotionally burdened. This renewed openness, typical of their pre-diagnosis relationship, enhanced their short amount of quality time.

Mr. Singer wanted to keep his job because the diversion was important to him (Thompson et al., 1993). Mrs. Singer wanted to stay home alone or with an aide. The social worker reintroduced the idea of adult day care, suggesting that Mrs. Singer could attend and assist the staff with other patients to the extent that she was able. Hesitantly, Mrs. Singer agreed to visit several adult day care centers with her daughter and husband. With Mrs. Singer's written permission, the social worker located a particularly inviting day care center where clients participated in interesting art projects. The staff was encouraging and open to Mrs. Singer's ideas. When she returned home that evening, she found herself thinking of ways to adapt art projects to various disabilities so more people could experience success. She decided she would attend only one day a week but, over time, increased her days at the center where the staff appreciated the talents she could still employ. Mrs. Singer felt useful and thought less about her disability and more about adapting art projects for the other center participants.

The Singers knew this stage of the disease could be very short, but they were able to enjoy the present. Occasionally, Mr. Singer would call the social worker to discuss his fear of the future. Together, they validated his fears and reminded each other that all anyone can count on is the moment.

Summary of the Counselor's Role

In this case, the first step for the social worker was interagency coordination between the Elder Care Center and the Visiting Nurses' Association. Once linkages were established and services were coordinated, the social worker was able to focus on the need for the couple to be helped to support each other. She used the safe, strong relationship she developed with the couple to help each of them to reach important goals. The social worker empowered Mrs. Singer by helping her to focus on her abilities rather than her increasing disability and, literally, helped her to find a role in which she had something valuable to contribute. Locating an adult day care center that understood Mrs. Singer's limitations and could use her artistic talents to help others was worth more to Mrs. Singer than hours of psychotherapy. The social worker empowered Mr. Singer by helping him to review the history of his marriage, validating his fears, giving him permission to be honest and open with his wife, and helping the couple to manage this tragedy together. As Mr. Singer's situation became more challenging, the social worker remained a safe and understanding haven for him. Throughout, she remained a resource for community services, an advocate and a counselor.

CONCLUSIONS

Several conclusions in regard to counseling the homebound can be drawn from the above case discussions. The first is that age is only one issue to consider in designing a plan for counseling. Frailty, illness and a resultant homebound state are the problems to be managed here. In fact, differences within age cohorts are more important in counseling than age. Also, the presence of dementia rather than the particular age of a person makes a dramatic difference in choice of effective counseling techniques. Dementia, in fact, changes everything; it is not only progressive and unremitting but it also does not allow the counselor to engage clients in ways that can empower them to help themselves.

As always in counseling, much of what transpires depends on a safe, respectful and trusting relationship between the counseling professional and clients. In this kind of work, it is always best to begin with concrete services; clients often require a specific service or apparatus and meeting concrete needs is a proven means of establishing trust. In fact, concrete services cannot be separated from counseling; each reinforces and each heightens the effect of the other.

No matter what other issues must be addressed in counseling the homebound elderly, loss in its various guises remains transcendent. In the most concrete sense, the homebound have lost mobility; they cannot leave the scene. People's worlds have shrunk to an apartment or sometimes to a room or a single chair. Other critical losses to be addressed relate to health, independence, financial security, important relationships, roles and a sense of control over their lives. In Mrs. Fredericks' situation, loss of control colored her view of self and decision making. Mr. and Mrs. Singer faced the loss of future. To move forward, Mrs. Broderick had to confront her mother's loss of the ability to reason and the loss of any possibility of attaining the kind of mother-daughter relationship for which she wished.

One continuing theme is that of helping the frail person and caregiver to weigh the wish for safety against the wish for autonomy. A related issue is the question of nursing home placement. No matter what the promise or contract between agency and individuals or between family members, the specter of having to live in a nursing home looms over each homebound situation. While in actuality it might ultimately be the safest and most comfortable solution, especially for an individual with advanced dementia, the nursing home represents the apotheosis of loss. Examples of the social, economic and emotional costs of nursing home placement can be seen in the cases of Mrs. Washington who manages to die at home, and Mrs. Madison who had to be placed in a nursing home.

Counseling involves work with several configurations of family members as well as work with individuals. In the four case examples, the social worker worked with mother and daughter, husband and wife, siblings and larger family units. Cases were chosen to demonstrate differences and similarities in counseling someone who lives by herself as opposed to someone living with others, counseling someone who is terminally ill as opposed to someone who does not face imminent death, counseling a family in which the ill person is dementing as opposed to helping a couple in which the ill spouse will remain intact mentally but will physically deteriorate and die usually within two years. Again, great skill is required in knowing how to work with family members separately and together so that each person feels cared for, understood and can support the primary client. Counseling requires the understanding of the family system and the patient and family's defense mechanisms so that the counselor can orchestrate his or her interventions. For example, the counselor may help a caregiver to deal with extended family members, remain socially active, address finances, and decide whether and/or when it is best for the ill individual to move to a nursing home. In turn, client and family caregivers must relate reasonably with professionals in order to get what they need, but for their ultimate growth and comfort, they have to attend to their relationships with each other. The examples of the Singers and Mrs. Crawford and Mrs. Madison attest to the importance of counseling in maintaining those salient relationships and helping them to mature.

In some situations, such as that of Mrs. Madison, the primary work is with the caregiver. In any case, the counselor addresses caregiver burden in helping to maintain a frail elderly person at home. Very old caregivers like Mrs. Washington's sister are often exhausted while middle-aged caregivers like Mrs. Broderick are pulled and stretched between husbands, children and families, jobs and parents. Some release, support and recreation outside the home remains important. In addition, the counselor always supports the relationship of primary client and caregiver since that relationship is probably most important to the homebound elderly person.

The mode of counseling that has been described for each of the cases is the best of clinical case management in that it employs sophisticated psychotherapy techniques and skills but does so without the rigidity or the protection of the traditional structure of psychotherapy (Kanter, 1989). Because boundaries in this kind of counseling are variable and loose, the counselor must be highly skilled in counseling techniques and in conscious use of self. An overarching counseling technique is supporting relational competence, making sure that clients maintain social relationships and social networks even in homebound status. This was illustrated in the social worker helping Mrs. Washington to resume her relationship with her minister, encouraging Mrs. Fredericks to maintain a relationship with the battered women's shelter and in locating an adult day care center which was an excellent match for Mrs. Singer.

One powerful set of tools in working with the homebound is reminiscence and lifetime review (Kaminsky, 1984; Norris, Stephans and Kinney, 1990). These techniques were very helpful to Mrs. Washington and Mr. Singer. They can be used in several ways. First, they can help the counselor assess how clients have dealt with troubling situations previously and understand that the homebound were not always the way that they appear in the present, that they looked different, could keep house differently and had richer social lives. Second, such tools strengthen homebound people's sense of self by reminding them of how they have managed their lives and assisting them in redefining themselves in terms of social networks and happier times. In addition, they are means for addressing depression and even loneliness.

Overall, the counseling goal for the frail elderly is to support the highest level of independence that the client and caregivers desire and can safely maintain in ways that respect family relationships and the integrity of the homebound person. Attainment of that goal requires that the counselor be skilled in service linkage and in the modes of relationship work and use of self of highly skilled clinicians. The homebound elderly continue to have the ability to adapt, to gain self-knowledge and to mature. Their capacity for engagement and growth is unrelated to their degree of disability or homebound status.

REFERENCES

Abramson, J. S. (1988). Participation of elderly patients in discharge planning: Is self-determination a reality? *Social Work, 33,* 443-448.

Barusch, A. S. (1988). Problems and coping strategies of elderly spouse caregivers, *The Gerontologist, 28,* 677-685.

Beaver, M. L. (1991). Life review/Reminiscent therapy. In Kim, P. K. H. (Ed.), *Serving the elderly: Skills for practice,* pp. 67-88. New York, NY: Aldine deGruyter.

Beckett, J. O. and Dungee-Anderson, D. (1989). Older minorities: Social work perspective. In Schneider, R. L. and Kropf, N. P. (Eds.), *Essential knowledge and skills for baccalaureate social work students in gerontology,* pp. 136-183. Washington, DC: Council on Social Work Education.

Brakman, S. V. (1994). Adult daughter caregivers, *The Hastings Center Report, 24,* 26-28.

Brown, J. C. (1990). Loss and grief: An overview and guided imagery intervention model, *Journal of Mental Health Counseling, 12,* 434-445.

Bulcroft, K., Kielkoph, M. R. and Tripp, K. (1991). Elderly wards and their legal guardians: Analysis of county probate records in Ohio and Washington, *The Gerontologist, 31,* 156-164.

Butler, R. N. (1974). Life review therapy: Putting memories to work, *Geriatrics, 29,* 165-173.

Butler, R. N., Lewis, M. and Sunderland, T. (1991). *Aging and mental health: Positive psychosocial and biomedical approaches* (4th ed.). New York, NY: Merrill.

Candib, L. M. (1994). Self-in-relation theory: Implications for women's health. In Dan, A. J. (Ed.), *Reframing women's health: Multidisciplinary research and practice*, pp. 67-78. Thousand Oaks, CA: Sage.

Coleman, P. G. (1986). *Aging and reminiscence processes: Social and clinical implications*. New York, NY: Wiley.

Compton, B. R. and Galaway, B. (1994). *Social work processes*. Pacific Grove, CA: Brooks/Cole.

Cox, E. O. and Parsons, R. J. (1992). Senior-to-senior mediation service project, *The Gerontologist*, 32, 420-422.

Cox, J. C. (1992). Objects of our affection, *SelfCare Journal*, p. 20.

Davis, J. H. (1987). Implications of the human-animal-companion bond in the community, *The Latham Letter*, Spring, 10-12.

Dossey, L. (1985). *Beyond illness: Discovering the experience of health*. Boston, MA: New Science Library.

Dossey, L. (1994). *Healing words: The power of prayer and the practice of medicine*. San Francisco, CA: Harper.

Dura, J. R., Stunkenberg, K. W., and Kiecolt-Glaser, J. K. (1991). Anxiety and depressive disorders in adult children caring for demented parents, *Psychology and Aging*, 6, 467-473.

Ganzer, C. and England, S. E. (1994). Alzheimer's care and service utilization: Generating practice concepts from empirical findings and narratives, *Health and Social Work*, 19, 174-181.

Gatz, M., Bengtson, V. L. and Blum, M. J. (1990). Caregiving families. In Bitten, J. E. and Schaie, K. W. (Eds.), *Handbook of the psychology of aging* (3rd ed., pp. 404-425). San Diego, CA: Academic Press.

Getzel, G. (1982). Group work with kin and friends caring for the elderly, *Social Work with Groups*, 5, 91-102.

Gilgun, J. F. (1994). An ecosystemic approach to assessment. In Compton, B. R. and Galaway, B. (Eds.), *Social work processes*, pp. 380-394. Pacific Grove, CA: Brooks/Cole.

Goldstein, H. (1983). Starting where the client is, *Social Casework*, 64, 267-275.

Gonyea, J. and Silverstein, N. (1991). The role of Alzheimer's disease support groups in families' utilization of community services, *Journal of Gerontological Social Work*, 16, 44-55.

Greene, R. R. and Lewis, J. S. (1990). Curriculum for case management with the frail elderly: A Delphi study, *Arete*, 15, 32-45.

Greene, V. L. and Monahan, D. J. (1989). The effect of a support and education program on stress and burden among family caregivers to frail elderly persons, *The Gerontologist*, 29, 472-477.

Gubrium, J. (1991). *The mosaic of care: Frail elderly and their families in the real world*. New York, NY: Springer.

Hansson, R. O. and Carpenter, B. N. (1994). *Relationships in old age: Coping with the challenge of transition*. New York, NY: Guilford.

Hansson, R. O., Remondet, J. H. and Galusha, M. (1993). Old age and widowhood: Issues of personal control and independence. In Stroebe, M. S., Stroebe, W.

and Hansson, R. O. (Eds.), *Handbook of bereavement: Theory, research and intervention*, pp. 367-380. Cambridge, England: Cambridge University Press.

Hennessy, C. H. (1989). Autonomy and risk: The role of client wishes in community-based long-term care, *The Gerontologist*, 29, 633-639.

Hooyman, N. R. and Kiyak, H. A. (1988). *Social gerontology: A multidisciplinary perspective*. Boston: Allyn and Bacon.

Iris, M. (1988). Guardianship and the elderly: A multi-perspective view of the decision making process, *The Gerontologist*, 28 (Suppl.), 39-45.

Hartman, A. (1994). Diagrammatic assessment of family relationships. In Compton, B. and Galaway, B. (Eds.), *Social work processes*, pp. 153-165. Pacific Grove, CA: Brooks/Cole.

Hashimi, J. (1991). Counseling older adults. In Kim, P. K. H. (Ed.), *Serving the elderly: Skills for practice*, pp. 33-49. New York, NY: Aldine deGruyter.

Jackson, B. (1993). *The caregivers' roller coaster: A practical guide to caregiving for the frail elderly*. Chicago, IL: Loyola University Press.

Kaminsky, M. (Ed.). (1984). *The uses of reminiscence: New ways of working with older adults*. New York, NY: The Haworth Press, Inc.

Kanter, J. S. (1989). Clinical case management: Definition, principles, components, *Hospital and Community Psychiatry*, 40, 361-368.

Kauffman, S. R. (1986). *The ageless self: Sources of meaning in later life*. Madison, WI: University of Wisconsin Press.

Keith, P. M. and Wacker, R. R. (1994). *Older wards and their guardians*. Westport, CT: Greenwood.

Kent, K. (1990). Elders and community mental health centers, *Generations*, 14, 19-21.

Kerson, T. S. (1989). *Social work in health settings: Practice in context*, New York, NY: The Haworth Press, Inc.

Kerson, T. S. (1989). Women and aging: A clinical social work perspective. In Garner, J. D. and Mercer, S. O. (Eds.), *Women as they age: Challenge, opportunity and triumph*, pp. 123-147. New York, NY: The Haworth Press, Inc.

Kerson, T. S. and Kerson, L. A. (1985). *Understanding chronic illness*. NY: Free Press.

Kerson, T. S. and Zelinka, J. D. (1989). Discharge planning: Acute medical service. In Kerson, T. S. (Ed.), *Social work in health settings: Practice in context*, pp. 195-212. New York, NY: The Haworth Press, Inc.

Labrecque, M. S., Peak, T., and Toseland, R. W. (1992). Long term effectiveness of a group program for caregivers of frail elderly veterans, *American Journal of Orthopsychiatry*, 62, 575-588.

Lowy, L. (1985). *Social work with the aging: The challenge and promise of the later years* (2nd ed.). New York, NY: Longman.

McCallion, P., Toseland, R. W., and Diehl, M. (1994). Social work practice with caregivers of frail older adults, *Research on Social Work Practice*, 4, 64-88.

Meen, R. (1987). Pets and mental health, *People-Animals-Environment*, pp. 21-25.

Mercer, S. O. and Robinson, B. (1989). Alzheimer's disease: Intervention in a nursing home environment. In Kerson, T. S. (Ed.), *Social work in health settings: Practice in context*, pp. 411-429. New York, NY: The Haworth Press, Inc.

Merriam, S. B. (1989). The structure of simple reminiscence, *The Gerontologist*, 29, 761-767.

Michelsen, R. W. (1989). Hospital based case management for the frail elderly. In Kerson, T. S. (Ed.), *Social work in health settings: Practice in context*, pp. 431-448, New York, NY: The Haworth Press, Inc.

Mohide, E. A., Pringle, D. M., Streiner, D. L., Gilbert, J. R., Muir, G., and Tew, M. (1990). A randomized trial of family caregiver support in the home management of dementia, *Journal of American Geriatrics Society*, 38, 446-454.

Morgan, D. L. (1982). Failing health and the desire for independence: Two conflicting aspects of health care in old age, *Social Problems*, 30, 40-50.

Morrow-Howell, N. (1992). Clinical case management: The hallmark of gerontological social work, *Journal of Gerontological Social Work*, 18, 119-131.

Myers, S. S. and Benson, H. (1992). Psychological factors in healing: A new perspective on an old debate, *Behavioral Medicine*, 18, 4-11.

Norris, V. K., Stephens, M. A. P., and Kinney, J. M. (1990). The impact of family interactions on recovery from stroke: Help or hindrance? *The Gerontologist*, 30, 535-542.

Overholser, J. C. (1991). The use of guided imagery in psychotherapy: Modules for use with passive relaxation training, *Journal of Contemporary Psychotherapy*, 21, 159-172.

Pearlman, D. N. and Crown, W. H. (1992). Alternative sources of social support and their impacts on institutional risk, *The Gerontologist*, 32, 527-535.

Perls, F., Hefferline, R., and Goodman, P. (1951). *Gestalt therapy: Excitement and growth in the human personality.* New York, NY: Dell.

Polster, E. and Polster, M. (1974). *Gestalt therapy integrated.* New York, NY: Vintage.

Proctor, E. and Davis, L. E. (1994). The challenge of racial difference: Skills for clinical practice, *Social Work*, 39, 314-321.

Raiff, N. R. (1993). *Advanced case management: New strategies for the nineties.* Newbury Park, CA: Sage.

Rathbone-McCuan, E. (1991). Family counseling: An emerging approach in clinical gerontology. In Kim, P. K. H. (Ed.), *Serving the elderly: Skills for practice*, pp. 51-66. New York, NY: Aldine deGruyter.

Roberto, K. A. (1992). Coping strategies of older women with hip fractures: Resources and outcomes, *Journal of Gerontology: Psychological Sciences*, 47, P21-P26.

Rodin, J. and Timko, C. (1992). Sense of control, aging, and health. In Ory, M. G., Abeles, R. P., and Lipman, P. D. (Eds.), *Aging, health and behavior*, pp. 174-206. Newbury Park, CA: Sage.

Rothman, J. (1994). *Practice with highly vulnerable clients: Case management and community based service.* Englewood Cliffs, NJ: Prentice-Hall.

Rubenstein, R. (1989). Themes in the meaning of caregiving, *Journal of Aging Studies*, 5, 119-130.

Saleeby, D. (1994). Culture, theory, and narrative: The intersection of meanings in practice, *Social Work*, 39, 351-359.

Salamon, M. J. (1986). *A Basic Guide to Working with Elders*. New York, NY: Springer.

Schlossberg, N. K. (1990). Training counselors to work with older adults, *Generations*, 14, 7-10.

Simos, B. (1979). *A Time to Grieve*. New York, NY: Family Service Society of America.

Skaff, M. M., and Pearlin, L. I. (1992). Caregiving: Role engulfment and the loss of self, *The Gerontologist*, 32, 656-664.

Smyer, M. A., Zarit, S. H. and Qualls, S. H. (1990). Psychological intervention with the aging individual. In Birren, J. E. and Schaie, K.W. (Eds.), *Handbook of the psychology of aging* (3rd ed.), pp. 375-403. San Diego, CA: Academic Press.

Soskis, C. W. and Kerson, T. S. (1992). The patient self determination act: Opportunity knocks again, *Social Work in Health Care*, 16, 1-18.

Teitelman, J. L. and Priddy, J. M. (1988). From psychological theory to practice: Improving frail elders' quality of life through control-enhancing interventions, *Journal of Applied Gerontology*, 7, 298-315.

Tennstedt, S. L., McKinlay, J. B., and Sullivan, L. M. (1989). Informal care for frail elders: The role of secondary caregivers, *The Gerontologist*, 29, 677-683.

Thompson, E. H., Futterman, A. M., Gallagher-Thompson, D., Rose, J. (1993). Social support and caregiving burden in family caregivers of frail elders, *Journals of Gerontology*, 48, S245-S254.

Talbott, M. M. (1990). The negative side of the relationship between older widows and their adult children: The mothers' perspective, *The Gerontologist*, 30, 595-603.

Tobin, S. S. (1991). *Personhood in advanced old age: Implications for practice*. New York, NY: Springer.

Toseland, R. W. , Rossiter, C. M., and Labrecque, M. S. (1989). The effectiveness of two kinds of support groups for caregivers, *Social Service Review*, 63, 415-432.

Toseland, R. W., Rossiter, C. M., Peak, T., and Smith, G. C. (1990). Comparative effectiveness of individual and group interventions to support family caregivers, *Social Work*, 35, 209-217.

Walker, A. J., Martin, S. S. K., and Jones, L. L. (1992). The benefits and costs of caregiving and care receiving for daughters and mothers, *Journal of Gerontology: Social Sciences*, 47, S130-S139.

Wallace, J. B. (1992). Reconsidering the life review: The social construction of talk from the past, *The Gerontologist*, 32, 120-128.

Weinberger, R. (1991). Teaching the elderly stress reduction, *Journal of Gerontological Nursing*, 17, 23-27.

Woods, M. E. and Hollis, F. (1990). *Casework: A psychosocial therapy* (4th ed.). New York, NY: McGraw-Hill.

Yeatts, D. E. (1992). Service use among low income minority elderly: Strategies for overcoming barriers, *The Gerontologist*, 32, 24-32.

York, D. E. (1994). *Cross cultural training programs.* Westport, CT: Greenwood.

Zarit, S. H. (1990). Interventions with frail elders and their families: Are they effective and why? In Stephens, M. A. P., Crowther, J. H., Hobfoll, S. E. and Tennenbaum, D. L. (Eds.), *Stress and coping in later-life families*, pp. 241-265. Washington, D.C.: Hemisphere.

Zook, E. (1992). A consideration of the role of care partners in long term care for the frail elderly, *Journal of Long Term Home Health Care*, 11, 27-34.

Chapter 9

Challenges for the Home Care Supervisor

Ann Burack-Weiss, DSW
Lucy Rosengarten, ACSW

INTRODUCTION

Supervision–the very word creates uneasiness, associated as it is with authority, responsibility, judgment–evaluation by a powerful "other." Literally meaning oversight, supervision may cause as much discomfort in the supervisor as in the supervisee; especially when the former is trained in one of the helping professions. How much does a supervisor have a right to expect from others? How can she balance the needs of those she supervises with the demands of those who supervise her?

In home care, the supervisor is accountable to the agency for assurance that service is being delivered in keeping with administrative directives. Timely completion of what is generally regarded as excessive paperwork is a crucial part of the job. Reimbursement from outside funders, as well as inter and intra-agency coordination, is dependent upon it.

At the same time, the supervisor is responsible to the home care client and his family caregivers for provision of service that enhances quality of life as well as performance of activities of daily living.

[Haworth co-indexing entry note]: "Challenges for the Home Care Supervisor." Burack-Weiss, Ann, and Lucy Rosengarten. Co-published simultaneously in *Journal of Gerontological Social Work* (The Haworth Press, Inc.) Vol. 24, No. 3/4, 1995, pp. 191-211; and: *New Developments in Home Care Services for the Elderly: Innovations in Policy, Program, and Practice* (ed: Lenard W. Kaye) The Haworth Press, Inc., 1995, pp. 191-211. Single or multiple copies of this article are available from The Haworth Document Delivery Service [1-800-342-9678, 9:00 a.m. - 5:00 p.m. (EST)].

© 1995 by The Haworth Press, Inc. All rights reserved.

Finally, the supervisor is responsible to her supervisees for training, consultation, and ongoing support. The home care supervisor may supervise case managers or be in a peer supervisory position with other agency professionals; however, the home care aide generally needs the most ongoing involvement.

The supervisor cannot favor one of the three functions at the expense of the others. She must perform a balancing act, mediating among these constituencies–interpreting each to the others, and, always maintaining her own equilibrium and professional role. These are the challenges facing the home care supervisor.

This chapter addresses the administrative, service, and training responsibilities of the home care supervisor under separate headings in order to highlight underlying principles. In practice, all three sets of responsibilities are often fulfilled through one intervention, as the case vignettes will illustrate. Although discussion is focussed on supervision of the home care aide, underlying principles and techniques are applicable to other paraprofessional home care workers as well.

The examples of supervisory practice used in this discussion are drawn from the procedural guidelines and client charts of a nonprofit home care agency in New York City, COHME, Inc. (Concerned Homemakers for the Elderly). Although many who read this chapter will find differences between COHME's organization and that of their own agency, the authors believe that the presentation of this model will suggest strategies that can be incorporated into a variety of settings.

About COHME

COHME was founded in 1985 by a geriatric social worker with 10 years experience as a line social worker in an urban, hospital-based certified home health care agency. COHME, licensed by the New York State Department of Health, is nonprofit and cooperatively organized. Its principles of organization are based on the founder's one year study of a successful home care agency in Bologna, Italy–a socialistic community where cooperativism is a way of life.

Although it has been difficult to adapt some aspects of Bologna's cooperativism to New York City's predominantly capitalistic culture, many features of cooperativism have been incorporated into policies affecting home health care workers, the aides who COHME calls home managers. Indeed, COHME's mission is two-fold: to provide excellent jobs for its workers and to provide excellent home care to frail and sick elderly.

Most home care supervision at COHME is performed by a professional (MSW) social worker who serves as case manager and team coordinator–with overall responsibility for the case. RNs and administrative staff often have important supervisory duties as directed by the MSW.

ADMINISTRATION

There are many agency variables that influence the job performance of the home care supervisor. Because she may have been (and probably was) trained as a clinician and learned what she knows of supervision on-the-job, she must become familiar with current theories of case management (Austin, 1983; Kaye, 1992; Downing, 1985; Silverstone and Burack-Weiss, 1983; Rothman, 1994).

The constraints of space allow discussion of only three agency variables: organizational structure, marketing/outreach, and recording requirements. The ways in which COHME integrates these administrative functions into the achievement of its mission to serve both clients and workers widens the parameters of possibility.

Organizational Structure

Most publicly-funded home care agencies can't afford the professional personnel necessary to do comprehensive MSW case manager/supervisor work. Medicare-funded certified agencies provide for limited MSW home visiting for the two to three months the client is on the acute care program. However, this MSW is a minor player in overall planning for the patient/client or for the agency. Medicaid-funded agencies are frequently overwhelmed. They may provide some social services performed by caring individuals who have no formal social work training. Community social work and nursing agencies, funded by a variety of public and private sources, have the potential commitment and personnel to do excellent case manager/supervisor work, but often their caseloads are too large and burnout or limited involvement may occur.

COHME is a nonprofit agency funded mainly by fee-for-service. It also received some small grants and contributions.

Professional geriatric care managers, usually MSWs or RNs, handle many case manager/supervisory tasks for a separate fee that is often nonreimbursable by government or insurance programs. They are frequently solo practitioners whose freedom from agency affiliation can have both positive and negative consequences for professional service delivery.

At COHME traditional attitudes about home manager supervision are often modified in the interest of limiting bureaucracy; still professional expertise is needed, recognized, and valued.

The nurse is responsible for all health-related problems arising in the home care situation. They are responsible for interviewing potential new home managers, preparing and giving in-service trainings related to nursing issues, making home visits or calling home managers into the office when immediate nursing information must be conveyed or work performance needs to be evaluated or altered, and being available to all staff whenever problems require nursing expertise.

Although nursing assessment is essential, the vision of the agency is founded on social work principles, and the professional MSW social worker is the home manager's primary supervisor. Home managers are home health aides with high school educations who go through an extensive testing and screening process by COHME's nurses and social workers.

At COHME, the social worker who functions as the *overall* manager of the case is called the case management team coordinator (CMTC). The CMTC's task is to gather information from the RN, physical therapist, home manager, administrative staff, and other members of the client's formal and informal system, including the client herself, for the purpose of creating an efficient assessment and care plan. She is the one responsible for selecting a home manager whose personality is compatible with that of the client and of negotiating with the client the number of hours per week that are necessary. The CMTC remains actively involved for the duration of the case, reviewing the entire chart and speaking with the client and others involved in the case at least once a week. The number of home visits, depending on the CMTC's assessment of the client's needs and on changes that occur as the case evolves, range from daily during crises to several times a year. She provides on-the-job supervision and support to the aide as well as working with informal system (family, friends, neighbors), coordinating efforts with other members of the COHME team. One CMTC can handle 20-25 clients with their home managers, depending on the intensity of the case management needed. As the census increases, more CMTCs are hired; her caseload does not increase.

COHME views every member of the staff, regardless of discipline or tasks, as a manager; that is to say, every member has an area of autonomy and contributes to the overall case plan. The CMTC mediates any differences that arise and interprets the needs of the client, family, and home manager to other members of the team. In the case that follows, everyone in the office has the potential to have a role in the overall case plan.

Case Example

> Mrs. P. called the business manager each Friday afternoon at 3:00 for a half-hour discussion of her bill prior to making out her check. The business manager had learned from the CMTC that accounting concerns were secondary to Mrs. P.'s need to demonstrate knowledge of money matters and control over her finances. Because of this he did not regard her call as an intrusion on his regular work; rather he saw it as a part of his regular work. Knowledge of the client and appreciation of his own unique role in preserving her self-esteem assisted him in "managing" his part of the case.

The home manager is expected to call into the office, every day she is on a case, and to keep narrative notes in "the yellow book" for review by the CMTC, client and family. These notes cover medications taken, the client's activities, and any other observations that seem noteworthy. Clients who do not have touch-tone phones are given phone adapters, to insure that home managers are able to access the agency's beeper system in emergency situations. The reason for this administrative directive is evident even in routine situations.

Case Example

> The CMTC was concerned about a client, Mr. M. Fearing that he would have trouble managing without her while she went on vacation, she advised the covering social workers to pay special attention to the case. When the CMTC returned, Mr. M. was the first client she asked about. The covering worker responded that Mr. M. had hardly noticed her absence; it was the home manager who had beeped her several times, needing the opportunity to share Mr. M.'s foibles and receive the CMTC's advice and support, who had truly missed her.

Because the CMTC cannot always take these calls immediately, the office manager assumes a central role; she becomes the "friendly voice" that insures home managers that they are part of a team—even when they feel isolated behind closed doors.

Marketing/Outreach

The case manager looks outside the agency not only for help for present clients but for referrals of potential clients. This can be a learning experience for the social worker who has worked at a line level in a nonprofit agency with little knowledge of the outreach or marketing energies needed to enable any such agency to survive. Although COHME receives some funding, its hybrid nature as a nonprofit agency that charges fees for its home managers, but charges nothing extra for its intensive case management, makes its financial needs difficult for traditional funders to understand. COHME must, therefore, be cooperative in its inside organization, but competitive with the many nonprofit and for-profit home care agencies that have mushroomed in the last 10 years. It does this not by telling–but by showing–the value of focused home care planning, a strategy that would work as well in providing outreach in underserved areas.

Case Example

The hospital social worker wanted action right away: "I have to get Mr. C. discharged tomorrow, with full time help. I have no time to wait." The CMTC arranged a visit at the patient's bedside two hours late–herself, the RN, two family members, the family lawyer and the hospital social worker. A good plan was worked out in one hour with the CMTC and COHME RN stopping the attending MD and floor RN for medical information as they rushed by. A home manager was on the way to the hospital by the interview's end, to meet the patient and family. The hospital social worker was pleased: "How'd you get so many people to work together so fast?" The CMTC explained that she's always coordinating home care services by bringing concerned people together, making assessments and plans, and bringing in community agencies. She and the COHME RN also had a lot of experience dealing with hospital pressures. The hospital social worker said she'd keep COHME in mind for her next difficult discharge. "We could handle less difficult situations too, you know," the CMTC said. Everyone smiled.

Recording Requirements

At COHME, documentation of services provided does more than fulfill mandated requirements. It is integrally bound to the provision of services. Client charts, called Black Books, contain all the paperwork related to a case. Although the office manager sometimes takes over these responsibilities due to time pressures, weekly review by the CMTC is the ideal.

Case Example

The CMTC had an unusual run of emergencies and a month elapsed before she had time to review the chart of Mrs. K. who was receiving 20 hours a week of home manager assistance while recovering from eye surgery. The case was stable and the review seemed routine, yet CMTC immediately noticed something troubling: the person designated as Mrs. K.'s primary physician had not responded to a request for medical information mailed two months earlier. The CMTC knew that there had once been two eye surgeons involved, and in a review of the narrative notes of the home manager (also in the black book) noted that the client was still visiting *both* eye surgeons. A follow-up call to the home manager revealed that the MD who had not returned the COHME letter was retired but still prescribing medicines for Mrs. K. which she was taking without the knowledge of the second doctor. The CMTC, recognizing the potential for confusion with medications, asked the RN to make a home visit to check all Mrs. K.'s medicines, speak to both MDs and coordinate care. She then sent out a new letter to the active MD and changed the name of the MD on the referral sheet, coverage sheet, and other pertinent pages.

DIRECT SERVICE TO CLIENTS AND FAMILIES

Provision of a quality, cost-effective service to clients and families is, of course, the driving principles of a home care agency. To accomplish this objective, the case manager/supervisor must: seek and mobilize client strengths, promote the optimum level of functioning possible, and provide the least restrictive environment–all the while respecting client diversity, confidentiality and dignity. These professional values must then be incorporated into a broad-based assessment of the individual client's physical, psychological, and social state, the setting of appropriate goals, and decisions about which interventions will best lead to achievement of those goals.

Sometimes one agency cannot meet all of the direct service needs of clients and families. In these cases the CMTC builds a geriatric team in the community–augmenting COHME services through collaboration with certified home care agencies (such as The Visiting Nurse Society or a hospital-based unit), allied health professionals (such as RNs, PTs, OTs), and home health aides. Professional geriatric care managers may also be called upon when a family's need for ongoing attention exceeds the norm that COHME is able to provide.

Assessment and Case Planning

Professional values, knowledge, and skills are necessary but not sufficient conditions for performing all the steps that lead to a successful care plan. The case manager/supervisor must possess an understanding of the aging process and be particularly sensitive to issues of pain and loss. Those who can no longer see, hear, think, or move as well as they once did; those who mourn losses of significant others who can never be replaced, often act out their feelings of anger and sorrow by making inappropriate demands of the home manager or agency. Then again, there are clients and family who are more content than they should be with the status quo; they need help in identifying environmental and social obstacles that stand in the way of their elders living life as fully as they are capable of doing.

Home care clients are often referred to as a "vulnerable" or "at risk" population, characterizations that say more about the limitations of society to accommodate their needs than about these needs themselves. Although dependence in activities of daily living propels many elders into home care, this dependence is hardly ever total, much less permanent. Strengths and inner resources acquired over a lifetime may be temporarily lessened by illness but they can often be restored with the support and encouragement of caregivers. Assistance in the performance of activities of daily living are the mainstay of home care; however, the case manager/supervisor should be cognizant of the psychosocial as well as practical aspects of client assessment and planning (Kane, 1987; Silverstone and Burack-Weiss, 1983, Burack-Weiss, 1988; Kirschner and Rosengarten, 1982; Kaye, 1992).

COHME uses a "One Sheet" for client assessment. It is filled out by the CMTC following *every* home visit. The clarity and brevity of this instrument forces the case manager/supervisor to discriminate between what is essential and what is of lesser importance in service to the individual client and to frame her plan in operational terms. The language makes it accessible to the home manager and administrative staff as well, facilitating their roles in the plan.

The "One Sheet" includes the following sections:

1. *Identifying Information* (I'm telling an objective story. "I just want the facts m'am.");

2. *Precipitating Event* (Why I'm involved now.);
3. *Assessment* (What I professionally think is happening and what needs to be done.); and
4. *Plan* (What I'm going to do.).

Intake

Most elderly and their families contact home care agencies at a time of crisis—previous methods of coping are no longer adequate and an immediate infusion of outside support is necessary. The following example illustrates the ways in which COHME's CMTC incorporates assessment skills into her response to a crisis situation. Note the role of the home manager as well; it will be elaborated on later in this chapter.

Case Example

Miss J. called COHME with an emergency situation. She was the only relative involved in the care of a childless aunt and uncle, Mr. and Mrs. E. Although Miss J. had received information about the agency's home care services some months ago (from a hospital social worker whom she had approached out of concern for her uncle's progressive Parkinson's disease) the aunt rejected help, preferring to do everything herself. Then, this morning, Miss J. was phoned by her distraught uncle who had awakened to find his beloved wife dead in the bed beside him. Neighbors were with him now, the niece reported, and she was on her way to her uncle's home to spend a night or two and prepare for Mrs. E.'s funeral. What could COHME do to help?

The CMTC obtained beginning referral information and arranged to meet the niece at Mr. E.'s home the following afternoon with a home manager. The CMTC selected a home manager whose personality she felt might be compatible with what she already knew about Mr. E. and who lived near him. She asked the RN to call Mr. E.'s MD for more medical knowledge.

Accompanied by the home manager and armed with the knowledge of a stable medical picture for Mr. E., the CMTC visited Mr. E. where she also met the niece, two caring neighbors and an old card-playing friend of Mr. E. The CMTC engaged them in a group meeting. Mr. E. was remarkably in control, though his speech and hearing were impaired and he often asked the niece to speak for him. Miss J. reported that Mr. E. had completely dressed and fed himself that morning, activities she had thought him incapable of doing without his wife's assistance. As conversation continued, the CMTC assessed that Mr. E. was exerting almost superhuman efforts to show everyone that he could manage for himself because he feared nursing home placement. She shared this assessment with the group, leading the niece to assure Mr. E. that he would remain at home. COHME was here for just this reason.

The CMTC encouraged the home manager to tell Mr. E. and the group what she could do to help him remain safely at home. The home manager, a young woman with an easy manner, knew Mr. E.'s neighborhood and needs. As she spoke in a reassuring fashion, Mr. E. began to cry, then stutter, then relax back in his chair. The group was concerned but the CMTC suggested that perhaps Mr. E. now felt safe enough to relax his guard and show his feelings of dependence and loss. Mr. E. agreed and slowly began to speak of his grief over the sudden death of his beloved wife.

After a time the CMTC toured the apartment with the niece while the home manager continued to speak with Mr. E., his neighbors and friend, gaining their trust. They found that the apartment was very clean but not at all adapted for disability. Various types of bathroom equipment were needed–tub seat, hand-held shower, grab bars, raised toilet seat as well as a medication box. The kitchen appliances were practically antique–working in quirky ways known only to Mrs. E. Together they discussed changes that would have to be made in the kitchen as well as medical equipment and assistive devices that would be ordered. The CMTC and home manager left the family group to continue to plan for the funeral. (To be continued on p. 207)

On-Going Service

The preceding case was perceived as a crisis situation by all involved; yet, many home care cases that lack its drama are felt to be crises by clients, families, or home managers. They, too, require an immediate response. Exploration, assessment, and intervention are apt to happen simultaneously. In every case the case manager/supervisor shares these tasks with the home manager.

The following incident, drawn from an on-going case, shows how potential flare-ups can be mediated and controlled by the astute case manager/supervisor.

Case Example

> The CMTC was confronted at her client's door by an angry home manager, "She wants me to wash windows! I'm not her maid!" The CMTC confirmed that yes, the client expected that; in fact the CMTC had, herself, cleaned the window on her first visit. The home manager who was new to the agency and new to the case was amazed. The CMTC went on to explain that for this client, unable to leave her studio apartment for weeks at a time, the window was "a window on the world"– and seeing through it was one of the few pleasures she had. Placing this task within the context of the overall case plan provided the necessary dignity that allowed the home manager to perform it with good grace.

(Of course, this incident could have been avoided if the home manager had been better-oriented to this client's special needs *before* arriving at the home. That is the agency ideal. In practice, however, a regular home manager can suddenly become ill or be otherwise unavailable and emergency replacement may not receive sufficient preparation in handling those idiosyncratic client needs that form the basis of a quality service. It is in situations such as these that the on-the-spot response of the CMTC can make or break the relationship between the elderly client and the home manager.)

TRAINING AND CONSULTATION

"The relationship to the teacher can be made stimulating, as well as protective, if it gives some picture of what fine accomplishment is, along with reassurance that one is not expected to meet it immediately" (Reynolds, 1965).

Bertha Reynolds said it first and best. The balance between demand and support is a crucial one for the case manager/supervisor to achieve. But she cannot stop there. She must have an understanding of adult learning in general and the special demands placed on it by the service needs of dependent clients. A basic understanding of supervisory principles in the human services is essential (Kadushin, 1985; Middleman and Rhodes, 1985; Rosengarten and Smith, 1990; Burack-Weiss and Brennan 1991).

Focus on the Home Manager

Case manager/supervisors do not direct the home manager's activities from afar; rather they are in constant contact with the home managers–partners in providing care. In order to do this successfully, they must be sensitive to the unique combination of assets and deficits that home care workers bring to the job.

Home managers, by and large, belong to disadvantaged sectors of society. The angry response of the home manager who was asked to wash windows typifies the resentment harbored by many who come to this work with a history of being exploited in low-paying, demeaning jobs. Because the income, education, language skills, and opportunity for advancement are generally lower for home managers than for others of the helping team, it is understandable that they may perceive certain housekeeping requests as assaults on their dignity. If we add to this mix the fact that more managers are often members of racial or ethnic minorities looked down upon by their clients, the imperative to direct attention to their needs is obvious.

The CMTCs at COHME recognize and accredit the special strengths that home managers bring with them. Many home managers come from cultural and religious backgrounds where caring for the elderly is valued. They appreciate the opportunity to be a "friend of the family," and the freedom from routinization that distinguishes home care from other jobs available to them.

At COHME, the CMTCs do in-home and in-office evaluations of home managers, which are always related to the home manager's assigned cases. They create and teach in-services, related to specific client or home manager problems. COHME RNs and guest speakers may also be called upon for their expertise in various fields.

In-Service Training

COHME pays home managers to attend four general meetings a year. These meetings combine administrative issues and in-service training. The twenty-five to thirty home managers who attend each meeting receive a light meal as well as an In-Service Award–important in building an "esprit de corps" and identification with the agency as well as contributing to feelings of professionalism.

The administrative portion of the meeting provides an opportunity to discuss agency-wide issues. Home manager participation is high as they realize that their complaints and suggestions are welcomed and acted upon.

At least 12 hours of in-service training a year are mandated by the New York State Department of Health. Some of these hours are fulfilled as part of the general meetings; the rest are covered by smaller group meetings held throughout the year and by attendance at relevant outside conferences.

Training sessions generally feature speakers or videos on topics decided upon by a joint committee of administrative staff and home managers. Trainings are always videotaped. These tapes and others on relevant topics are available to all through the COHME library; the library also circulates a large array of print materials and audio tapes.

Some trainings provide information about health-related problems and situations faced by COHME clients (incontinence, Alzheimer's disease, foot care, exercise needs); others provide insight into psychosocial issues (special needs of gay and lesbian clients, family caregiving, elder abuse); still others address interactional processes (building a trusting relationship, cooperativism in practice). COHME keeps these meetings lively and innovative. Dialogue with guest speakers from the community, and creative exercises underscore the participatory ethic of the agency.

COHME meets sensitive interactional problems head on. For example, in one training film "Developing a Trusting Relationship with your Home Care Client," potentially conflictual situations are presented and alternative ways of handling them are discussed. Conflict is usually due to the fact that the client is white and the worker is black. The home managers are eager to express their thoughts and feelings about racial stereotypes and to discuss their concerns regarding being perceived by clients as servants rather than home managers. Then, in an effort to bridge the gap between client and worker, similarities in their conditions are identified: women's issues, financial worries, problems with children, and family stresses are common concerns. Finally, the home managers see that acceptance by society is an issue for both the elderly and people of color.

In recognition of the fact that attitudinal change does not automatically translate into changes in action–practical "how to" advice is given. In working with the "difficult client," for example, home managers are urged never to say things like 'relax.' They are asked what client feelings might be behind the difficult behavior (fear of confinement? loneliness?). As they gain perspective, home managers are helped to develop their own coping strategies. In dealing with the angry client, for example, the home manager is encouraged to put up a mental screen. "You can see through the screen but the words don't directly hit you." Ask: (1) "Why is Mrs. O. treating me this way?" Say: (2) "I'm a professional, she's ill and my client, I'm not going to take it personally." But: (3) "I'm not going to be condescending or patronizing; I'll be charitable and compassionate."

At COHME, the development and reworking of in-service training curriculum is constant. Trainings about working with clients with dementia are a case in point. Over time, these evolved from sessions focussing on the mentally impaired client to sessions focussing on how work with the mentally impaired client creates emotional stresses for the home manager. As home managers demonstrated their need to speak and be heard–to share their experience with peers in similar situations–COHME saw that a change in emphasis was needed.

Team Meetings

When a client is receiving total home manager care (168 hours weekly, with 3-4 home managers assigned to the case) a monthly group meeting, led by the CMTC, is held in the office. A trained substitute home manager is assigned to the client while this is going on.

These meetings not only help home managers identify and resolve client management issues sometimes obscured in the hustle and bustle of daily duties; they give home managers a special opportunity, in the quiet of the office setting, to raise problems they might have with the agency itself. This can require the CMTC to balance her supervisory and administrative roles.

Case Example

The first few monthly group (four home managers) meetings about Mrs. G's care, held by the CMTC in her private office with the door closed, were dominated by illness issues; the next three by how the many work tasks could be more fairly divided among the four home managers. By the seventh monthly meeting, major problems had been resolved. The CMTC and four workers knew each other well, style differences among the workers had been accepted, and a measure of comfort with casual conversation was achieved. Home managers began to ask questions about COHME's policies and procedures, their benefits, and the process by which work assignments were made. The CMTC, delighted at the participatory cooperative spirit the home managers had shown, brought their questions into the weekly administrative meetings. Administrative staff were not so delighted: home managers should come to them directly or ask their questions at general meetings, they believed. The CMTC agreed that general meetings would be a better forum, while pointing out that her small group meetings gave home managers the time to develop courage to raise their issues in a larger group. It was resolved that the CMTC would limit but not stifle discussion of administrative concerns. At the same time, she would explain to the home managers that she could not be their "middle man." She also considered having fewer supervisory group meetings whenever case-related issues had been resolved.

One-on-One Interventions

"Be secure enough to ask for help" is a framed COHME motto. "There's no such thing as a dumb question" is the verbal follow-up.

The case manager/supervisor–home manager relationship can be a difficult one to navigate. On the one hand, the supervisor wants to recognize the home manager's ability to act in a responsible, autonomous manner in situations that are within her domain. On the other hand, overestimating the home manager's ability may place a client at risk–as well as being detrimental to the home manager's self-esteem.

Case Example

(We continue with the case of Mr. E.) After that first meeting, the CMTC encouraged the home manager to advocate with the building superintendent for new kitchen appliances, enlisting the neighbors (with whom who she now felt comfortable) as advocates if she needed them. The home manager, successful in getting the appliances, was very proud of herself and received much praise from the agency. The CMTC also arranged for the RN to visit the home to assess and order the needed medical equipment and assistive devices. The RN was so impressed with the home manager's handling of the kitchen appliances that she simply left the list of needed items and the name of the medical supply company with the home manager and asked her to order them. The home manager called the company, but the order never went through. A surly clerk asked questions about Medicare and sizes that she didn't understand: she got flustered and anxious, hung up, and was ashamed to tell anyone. It was only when the articles did not arrive that the CMTC realized what had happened. First, she spoke to the RN–requesting that in the future she either order equipment herself or ask the office to do it. Then, she asked the home manager why she had not called her, or the office, for help. The home manager replied that she'd been so successful and knew COHME expected a lot from her. The busy RN's request seemed only a short extra step to take; however, she didn't understand what the clerk was talking about and it made her feel inadequate, frightened, and unprofessional. The CMTC assured her that she was an excellent home manager who had never been instructed on what she was asked to do–COHME was wrong to ask her to do a task before training her to do it. She then went on the underscore that the agency expects her to ask for help when it is needed.

Evaluation

COHME evaluates home managers yearly, in home and in the office. Hourly raises are tied to job performance. In preparation, the CMTC uses three methods of data collection: the home manager's personnel file, a home visit to a current case (that involves the client's opinions to the extent that he or she is able to participate), and an office meeting between the CMTC and the home manager. The personnel file consists of copies of positive or negative observations about the home manager made during daily to weekly entries by the CMTC into the black book. The two evaluation forms, developed by the agency over time, cover similar criteria: professional responsibilities, communication skills, dependability, initiative, cooperation, and administrative compliance. The difference lies in emphasis. The home visit is limited to the client–home manager relationship and the office visit includes the agency–home manager relationship. Both visits are scored on a Likert scale with performance ranging from outstanding to unsatisfactory. The office evaluation also includes a narrative summary that amplifies the checklists, provides a rationale for salary adjustment, and furnishes the agency with information valuable in making future assignments.

Evaluation Excerpts

"Ms. P. does tend to take control of situations; but on appropriate cases this is a wonderful trait."

"Ms. C. was on five difficult cases this year–besides clients being resistant (two with Alzheimer's disease) there were a multitude of family issues involved which made situations even more difficult. Despite this Ms. C. always seemed to make an effort to try her best, and when she sensed her limitations she would let us know."

"Ms. D. provided care to client in the hospital and was well able to serve as client's advocate in a chaotic situation."

Difficulties of the COHME Supervisory Paradigm

The COHME mission (to care as much for its workers as it does for its clients) highlights problems that exist to some degree in every home care agency.

The agency knows that well-trained, well-supervised, well-treated home managers will have higher self-esteem and translate the caring they receive from the CMTC and the rest of staff into giving better care to their elderly clients. It must be clearly recognized, however, that home managers often have long-standing personal problems that can hinder their job performance.

The case manager/supervisor may be supervising a competent and caring home manager who is functioning on a high enough level to give good care. She may assess that with social work counselling which she's eager to give, the home manager would be able, for example, to go back to school, handle a family problem, and have needed dental work done. It is understandable that the case manager/supervisor would want to help home managers improve their functioning; especially when she sees untapped potential. It's not a good idea.

First, there are agency constraints and priorities. There isn't time or reimbursement for the psychosocial counselling of home managers. Secondly, the home manager sees the supervisor as an agent of the agency that pays her. Sharing personal difficulties with someone who evaluates her professional performance places her in a vulnerable position. Most importantly, the home manager didn't come to the agency for personal counselling–but for a job. It should be recognized that a work-related or personal crisis is time-limited. If the home manager is not able to reach her prior level of functioning after referral to an appropriate community agency for counselling, she must be helped to go on leave until she works things out.

CONCLUSION

Home care is the most intimate of service settings. At its best, it can foster a loving bond forged by the hour-to-hour sharing of everyday life. At its worst, home care can lead to subtle and gross instances of abuse as client or home attendant act out their frustrations on one another. Home care situations are subject to rapid change. Client improvement or deterioration, home attendant on-the-job or off-the-job crises–all place demands on the case manager/supervisor for prompt action.

The ability of the home care supervisor to balance administrative, direct service and training/consultation responsibilities can make the difference between an elderly woman's remaining in the community or entering an institution, between an elderly man's feeling like a prisoner in his own home or continuing to feel like the master of his life. The ability of the home care supervisor also has significant consequences for the home manager–elevating what could be just another menial job into an important service of which she can be rightfully proud.

The presentation of a model runs the risk of sounding reductive. Case examples work out neatly. Team collaboration seems effortless. In fact, COHME is not immune to the problems that face every home care agency. The practice principles and COHME experience described here are, thus, presented as a work in progress–a point of departure for consideration for an area of gerontological practice that has not received adequate attention to date.

REFERENCES

Austin, C. (1983). "Case management in long term care: Options and opportunities," *Health and Social Work*, 8, 16-30.

Burack-Weiss, A. and Brennan, F.C. (1984). *First encounters between elders and agencies: A practice guide.* NY: Brookdale Institute on Aging and Adult Human Development, Columbia University.

Burack-Weiss, A. (1988). "Clinical aspects of case management," *Generations*, 23-29.

Burack-Weiss, A. and Brennan, F.C. (1991). *Gerontological social work supervision.* Binghamton, NY: The Haworth Press, Inc.

Downing, R. (1985). "The elderly and their families." In Weil, M. Karls and associates (Eds.), *Case management in human service practice.* San Francisco: Jossey-Bass.

Hasenfeld, Y. (1983). *Human service organizations.* Englewood Cliffs, NJ: Prentice Hall.

Kadushin, A. (1985). *Supervision in social work* (2nd ed.). NY: Columbia University Press.

Kane, R.A. (1987). "Comprehensive assessment." In Maddox, G.L. (Ed.), *The Encyclopedia of Aging.* NY: Springer.

Kaye, L.W. (1992). *Home health care.* Newbury Park, CA: Sage Publications, Inc.

Kirschner, C. and Rosengarten, L. (1982). "The skilled social work role in homecare," *Social Work.*

Middleman, R. and Rhodes, G. (1985). *Competent supervision.* Englewood Cliffs, NJ: Prentice Hall, Inc.

Reynolds, R.C. (1965). *Learning and teaching in the practice of social work.* Silver Spring, MD: NASW.

Rosengarten, L. and Smith, G. (1990). "Training aides in caring for persons with dementia." In *Pride Institute Journal of Long Term Home Health Care,* 9, 3 (Summer).

Rothman, J. (1984). *Practice with highly vulnerable clients: Case management and community-based service.* Englewood Cliffs, NJ: Prentice Hall.

Silverstone, B. and Burack-Weiss, A. (1983). *Social work practice with the frail elderly and their families: The auxiliary function model.* Springfield, IL.

Chapter 10

Clinical Assessment in Home Care

Miriam K. Aronson, EdD
Joanne Kennedy Shiffman, RNC, GNP

INTRODUCTION

There has been unprecedented growth in the number and proportion of elderly persons during the twentieth century. This increased
longevity is due in large measure to public health advances, such as
vaccination and treatment of infectious diseases. Additionally, there
has been increased survival by the elderly themselves due to improved medical management. This growth of the elderly population
and simultaneous dramatic growth of the very elderly, is projected
to continue well into the next century. Since the elderly as a population subgroup are the heaviest users of health services, these demographic trends have significant implications for formulation of
health and social policy (Aronson, 1994).

Accompanying current initiatives for control of escalating health
care costs for the elderly and disabled, there is an effort to move
services out of the most expensive institutional settings to alternative sites. There is also an attempt to shift costs from third-party
payors such as Medicare to the ill individuals themselves. As part of
this shift, home health care is becoming increasingly popular.

It was reported in a recent study that many elderly patients are

[Haworth co-indexing entry note]: "Clinical Assessment in Home Care." Aronson, Miriam K., and
Joanne Kennedy Shiffman. Co-published simultaneously in *Journal of Gerontological Social Work*
(The Haworth Press, Inc.) Vol. 24, No. 3/4, 1995, pp. 213-231; and: *New Developments in Home
Care Services for the Elderly: Innovations in Policy, Program, and Practice* (ed: Lenard W. Kaye)
The Haworth Press, Inc., 1995, pp. 213-231. Single or multiple copies of this article are available from
The Haworth Document Delivery Service [1-800-342-9678, 9:00 a.m. - 5:00 p.m. (EST)].

© 1995 by The Haworth Press, Inc. All rights reserved.   *213*

214 NEW DEVELOPMENTS IN HOME CARE SERVICES FOR THE ELDERLY

being discharged from hospitals earlier than in the past and are trying to avoid nursing home entry. As a result, the report said, older Americans "will pay 500 percent more out-of-pocket for home health care services in 1994 than in 1987," a staggering increase in out-of-pocket costs (American Association of Retired Persons, 1994). Another recent study revealed regional disparities in the utilization of home care services, with much more home health utilization in the northeast (National Health Provider Inventory, 1991). With the projected growth of the very elderly population subgroup nationwide, the demand for home care and other long-term care services will increase in all regions.

Impending cuts in Medicare and other entitlements will force elderly and disabled persons to compete for the available scarce resources and share an increasing proportion of the costs of health services. Methods of allocation will be of great concern to providers and consumers alike and it is inevitable that there will be increased attention focused on how home care needs are assessed.

STATE OF THE ART OF ASSESSMENT

There is no standardized assessment. Rather, current practice under the Medicare and Medicaid programs is for a physician to write orders for home care services. A nurse, social worker or allied health professional usually visits the home and evaluates the situation. After this assessment and a review of the doctor's orders, a care plan is developed. The level of assessment skill and the comprehensiveness of the plan vary from provider to provider, and the plan may be heavily influenced by the availability of reimbursement. The elderly and disabled, with their interacting multiple conditions and situations, often test the boundaries of reimbursement criteria.

As health care continues to be an issue of fiscal and public policy concern and as demands increase for home care, unanswered questions about cost and benefit will need to be addressed. Thus, there is increased pressure for development of a standardized methodology for determination of entitlements and measurement of outcomes. The Health Care Financing Administration (HCFA) is leading an effort to develop a multidimensional assessment tool for use with

Medicare home care recipients to determine needs and measure outcomes. An attempt has been underway for almost a decade, but there is currently renewed interest and activity in this regard.

Various states are also moving in the same direction, since they provide half of the budget for Medicaid, which supplies a significant amount of home and personal care services to the elderly and disabled. These attempts have not been without challenge. New York is a case example. In July, 1992, New York State implemented the Home Assessment Resource Review Instrument (HARRI) for purposes of assessing functional needs and determining service entitlements. The tool was developed to meet requirements of cost-containment imposed by state legislation. Its challengers describe it as "task-oriented and lacking individualization" and question its validity and reliability, since they say it was implemented without field testing. They also contend that it violates Medicaid and state law (Home Care Advisory Committee, Dowd v. Bane, 1993). Thus assessment for home care entitlements is an issue with implications that reach far beyond an individual household.

THE ASSESSMENT PROCESS

Because of their complex problems and needs, home care clients require a comprehensive assessment which must include data regarding: health status; physical functioning; cognition; mood and affect; environment; safety; social supports; and legal and financial issues. Input may be required from several different sources. Ideally, an assessment instrument would be able to quantify these various aspects of an individual's health and function for the purpose of developing a treatment plan and predicting outcomes.

Unfortunately, there is no single universal tool at this time although a number of multidimensional tools are available. These include the Older Americans Resources & Services instrument (OARS): Multidimensional Functional Assessment (Center for the Study of Aging and Human Development, 1978); the Comprehensive Older Persons Evaluation (COPE) (Pearlman, 1987); the Comprehensive Assessment & Referral Evaluation (CARE) (Gurland, Kuriansky, Sharpe, Simon, Stiller, and Burkett, 1977); and the Popovich scale (Popovich, Grubba, and Jirovec, 1990) (Table 1).

TABLE 1. Multidimensional Instruments

	Function Assessed	Administration	Utilization
Multidimensional Functional Assessment Questionnaire (OARS)	Measures functional status in the social, economic, mental health, physical health and ADL domains—and impact of alternative services.	Trained interviewers 1 hr. 105 items	Geared toward the elderly; with information specific to functioning and services.
Comprehensive Assessment & Referral Evaluation (C.A.R.E.)	Multidimensional tool assessing physical, mental, social, nutritional, and economic aspects; items of each domain scattered throughout interview to reduce stress.	Trained interviewers 45 min. - 1 1/2 hr.	Geared toward elderly both hospitalized and/or community; to measure functioning in that environment and examine changes in complaints or functioning over time.
Comprehensive Older Persons Evaluation (C.O.P.E.)	Assesses 8 areas with questions covering: legal, demographic, social, financial, physical, functional, and IADLs.	Trained interviewers 30 - 45 min. 28 items	Comprehensive general data base geared toward the elderly.
Popovich Scale	Assesses overall presentation of the patient, caregiver and environment in the home via 4 subscales: cognitive, economic, social, and physical domains.	R.N. 30 - 45 min. 28 items	Used in home-care; identifies patients and caregivers at risk for home care complication.

These instruments vary in level of comprehensiveness and complexity and applicability to home care. Several of the available tools were developed for research on community-based samples. Only the Popovich scale was developed for evaluating needs for home health care.

No matter what the assessment tool, there is no substitute for an assessor with good listening and observational skills. Sources of information for the assessment may include patient self-report, medical records, informant interview, and direct observation. Where there is a lack of an informant and a dearth of historical information or where inconsistencies in function are observed, the assessment may need to span a more extended period of observation. While considerable data may be available from hospital records and discharge planning personnel, a home visit increases the accuracy of assessment.

Every patient is a person with a personality and a sense of self. The intrinsic factors have been shaped by life experience. A good assessment must uncover this information in a sensitive, empathic fashion. Although the assessment process is described according to various domains, the client is *not* merely a diagnosis or organ system.

Health Status. It is important to ascertain diagnoses as well as information about severity, prognosis and functional impact. Not only is objective information about medical history necessary, but it is also advisable to query the patient's health beliefs and cultural background, as this will likely affect compliance. Additionally, a review of medications, including both prescription and over-the-counter drugs is needed. The assessor must always look for signs of alcohol or other substance abuse and also for indications of elder abuse.

Nutritional status must be noted, not only in terms of the patient's appearance and current weight but also in terms of previous status. The assessor must also look for evidence of ability to obtain or prepare food, e.g., What is in the refrigerator? Does the stove work?

Information about an individual's sleep patterns will heavily influence the scheduling of care and needs to be queried in the assessment process.

Instruments which are used to determine health status include the

Sickness Impact Profile (Bergner, Bobbitt, Pollard, and Gilson, 1976) and the Physical and Mental Health Questionnaire (Milne, Maule, Cormack, and Williamson, 1972) (Table 2).

Physical Functioning. Task performance has generally been used as the marker for physical functioning. Instruments have been developed to assess performance of the basic Activities of Daily Living (ADLs) such as bathing, dressing, toileting, grooming, feeding, and mobility. The importance of mobility must not be underestimated, as the ability to move around impacts all other activities. ADL abilities are regarded as necessary for independent function in the community. Commonly used ADL instruments include the Katz ADL Scale (Katz, Downs, Cash, and Grotz, 1965), the Barthel Index (Mahoney and Barthel, 1965), and the Kenny Self-Care Scale (Schoening and Iversen, 1968) (Table 3).

Other tools address the Instrumental Activities of Daily Living (IADL), such as handling finances, using a telephone, shopping, and traveling. Measures of IADLs include the Instrumental Activities of Daily Living (Lawton and Brody, 1969) and the Pfeffer Functional Activities Questionnaire (Pfeffer, Kurosaki, Harrah, Chance, and Filos, 1982) (Table 3).

Cognition. An individual's ability to function independently and safely is related to his/her intellectual abilities, especially in terms of memory, orientation, and judgment. Cognitive status also affects a patient's ability to supervise home services. In an elderly population, Alzheimer's and related dementias are the major causes of mental impairment. Since Alzheimer's and related dementias are age-dependent, the index of suspicion must be high when working with very elderly individuals (Aronson, Ooi, Geva, Masur, Blau, and Frishman, 1991). Cognitive impairment is a frequent primary condition as well as a comorbidity and its negative impact on the ability to survive independently must not be underestimated. Since many individuals with cognitive impairments have good social skills and may be able to cover their deficits in casual conversation, a mental status test should be included in all assessments.

There are several reliable and valid screening tools which can be administered in under ten minutes by a trained individual. While these tests are not diagnostic in and of themselves, they are good indicators of the presence and severity of cognitive impairment and

TABLE 2. Instruments Assessing Health Status

	Function Assessed	Administration	Utilization
Sickness Impact Profile	Health Status and sickness-related dysfunction, related to effect on 12 subscales of ADLs in multidimensional arena.	Respondent self-report 136 items	Performance-oriented functional status measure that occurs over time within an illness group.
Physical and Mental Health Questionnaire	Assessment of past and current medical health history; cognitive and emotional assessment and physical exam.	Registered Nurse/M.D. 30 min.	Physical health specific to certain disease entities, with assessment section for dementia/ and emotional/depressive illness.

TABLE 3. Instruments Assessing Physical Function

	Function Assessed	Administration	Utilization
Katz ADL Scale	Basic Self-Care: Bathing, Dressing, Toileting, Transfer, Continence, Feeding.	Interviewer 15 min.	Simple assessment of <u>basic</u> everyday skills; on a 6-level Guttman Scale ranging from Independent to Dependent.
Barthel Index	Self-Care and Ambulation.	Interviewer 25 min. +	Assessment of functional status including ambulation, w/c propulsion, & stair climbing—Weighted value with 100 points indicating independence on all items. Score reflects ability or inability to do personal care.
Instrumental ADL Scale	More complex activities; finances, dialing phone, shopping, self-medication, housekeeping.	Interviewer/observer 5 min.	Assesses function for independent living.
Kenny Self-Care Scale	Self-Care and Ambulation.	Interviewer 15-20 min.	Utilized in rehabilitation settings.
Functional Activities Questionnaire	Functional activities assessed by clinical tests done by patient.	Interviewer/Family Caregiver 15 min.	Distinguishes functional impairments and resulting states of dependency; sensitive to early changes in dementia.

can be used to track the progress of intellectual decline. Two of the most commonly used instruments are the Mini-Mental State Examination (MMSE) (Folstein, Folstein, and McHugh, 1975) and the Blessed Information-Memory and Concentration Test (IMC) (Blessed, Tomlinson, and Roth, 1968) (Table 4). When an individual scores in the impaired range and this condition represents a change in function, there is need for a diagnostic workup for dementing illness. In an individual with a diagnosed dementing illness, there must be adaptation of the care plan to accommodate the new level of deficits. For example, a disoriented patient cannot self-medicate (Agostinelli, Demers, Garrigan, and Waszynski, 1994) and may not be able to assure his/her own adequate food intake. While there are more in-depth dementia assessment tools, the burden of assessment must be considered in relation to the utility of the information obtained.

Dementia involves cognitive, functional, and behavioral impairments. Behavioral symptoms may include agitation, wandering, sleep-wake disturbances, paranoia, hallucinations, poor impulse control, verbal and physical aggression, sexual inappropriateness, apathy and depression (Aronson, 1994). These associated behaviors may strongly affect the feasibility of providing care in the home. For example, a wanderer cannot be left alone, and if 24-hour services are not available, institutionalization may become necessary. Individuals with dementia are generally not good historians, especially as related to their behavior problems and these may not be evident during a short interview. Therefore, the assessor must obtain information about behavior from the primary caregiver or other informants. Another caveat is that behaviors demonstrated during an acute hospitalization may not reflect the true functioning of the patient; thus assessment must be ongoing. Information about changes needs to be used to modify the care plan periodically.

Mood and Affect. Depression is a common comorbidity in medical illness and in dementia. Depression may impose an overlay of "excess disability" on already compromised function, thus increasing care requirements and decreasing quality of life. Because depression is a treatable illness, it is important for clinicians to diagnose and treat it. In the elderly, depression may be less obvious, since depressive symptoms may be masked or may present as

TABLE 4. Instruments Assessing Cognitive Function

	Function Assessed	Administration	Utilization
Folstein's Mini-Mental State Exam	Memory, orientation, attention, constructional ability.	Trained Interviewer 10 min. 2 parts - verbal and performance: 4 verbal sub-test with max. score 21 2 performance sub-test with max. score 9	Fairly quick and sensitive test; detecting moderate impairment.
Blessed Information-Memory and Concentration Test.	Memory, orientation, concentration, performance.	Trained Interviewer 25 min. 27 questions or verbal trials.	Differential diagnosis between functional and organic forms of mental disorders.

physical complaints, such as fatigue and sleep disturbance. Some of the more commonly used screening tools are the Geriatric Depression Scale (GDS) (Brink, Yesavage, Lum, Heersema, Adey, and Rose, 1982); the Zung Self-Rating Depression Scale (SDS) (Zung, 1965; McKegney, Aronson, and Ooi, 1985); the Philadelphia Geriatric Center Morale Scale (Lawton, 1975), the Depression Inventory (Beck and Beamesderfer, 1974) and the Hamilton Depression Inventory (Hamilton, 1967) (Table 5). These instruments are not diagnostic, but abnormal scores indicate a need for medical and/or psychiatric evaluation and follow-up. Which tool is selected is not as critical as the need to include depression screening in the clinical assessment. A history of other psychiatric conditions must be obtained as well.

Environment. One of the most important determinants of need for home health care is where an individual resides. Those elderly living alone are substantially more vulnerable to institutionalization, as their isolation and functional dependency put them substantially at risk. A comprehensive assessment needs to take into account the circumstances of the patient which would be supportive or detrimental to a particular treatment strategy. For example, are family members available to assure compliance with the care plan?

Safety is another critical issue. If an individual cannot be safe in his/her home, homecare may not be feasible. Extreme clutter may be a fire hazard as well as a risk factor for falling. A history of falling within the last six months may place an individual at greater risk for additional falls. Further, if an individual has an unsteady gait or difficulty transferring, going to the bathroom during the night unaided could put them at high risk for falling.

Social Supports. Social supports include informal supports such as family, friends and neighbors, as well as formal care providers. An older person's ability to remain in the community can be enhanced by informal assistance from a number of sources. For example, are there neighbors who shop, prepare meals, or provide transportation? Are there friends who do chores? Are there children who visit? The availability of informal supports may be underreported in an interview with the older person. A home visit often reveals evidence of informal helpers, e.g., visits, phone calls, chores. A good plan will mobilize existing social supports and provide ser-

TABLE 5. Instruments Assessing Emotional State

	Function Assessed	Administration	Utilization
Geriatric Depression Scale	Symptoms of Depression	Self or Interviewer 5 min. Short form-15 items Long form-30 items	Designed for elderly; broad questions regarding mood; quick; reliable.
Zung Self-Rating Depression Scale	Symptoms of Depression	Self Administration 5 min. 20 items	Simple format; focuses on somatic complaints.
Beck Depression Inventory	Symptoms of Depression	Self Administration 5 min. 21 items	Validated in elderly patients; focuses heavily on somatic complaints.
Hamilton Depression Inventory	Symptoms of Depression	Psychiatrist, Psychologist or Trained Health Professional 20 min. 21 items	Designed for adults of all ages; identifying factors of depression, anxious depression, and index of instability.
Philadelphia Geriatric Center Morale Scale	Symptoms of Depression	Self or Interviewer 5 min. 22 items	Designed for elderly; measures subjective well-being.

vices that are complementary and supplementary. Good communication with and support of the social supports must be incorporated into the practice of all home care providers.

Legal and Financial. Legal issues often surface during times of crisis, especially when dementia is a primary condition or a comorbidity. The ability to make decisions about important matters such as living arrangement, health care, and use of financial resources may be impaired, and this impairment may prevent the patient from getting needed services. Implementing a care plan may, therefore, be a juggling act since legal intervention is not the norm. Most individuals with dementia do not have court-appointed legal guardians. Therefore, an important part of some care plans may be to seek legal services to enable use of an individual's resources for their own care. Another important aspect of legal planning is to ascertain the existence of advanced directives such as designated health care representatives, living wills, Do Not Resuscitate orders, and wishes regarding artificial feeding and/or hydration.

Financial considerations are also key. Some individuals have sufficient private resources to meet their own needs. Others, however, must rely on external sources, such as community agencies and entitlements such as Medicare or Medicaid. All programs have their own sets of criteria and different levels of bureaucratic processes, so implementation may be subject to delays. To further complicate matters, many older persons are reluctant to divulge their finances, and simple determinations often cannot be made. Family members may or may not be helpful in this regard.

CULTURAL DIVERSITY

Another important aspect of planning for home health care services is cultural diversity. The elderly population is becoming more racially and ethnically diverse. Likewise, home health care providers themselves are a heterogenous group. The home health care workforce consists predominantly of disadvantaged women, with a substantial representation of minorities (Hollander-Feldman, Sapienza, and Kane, 1990).

This diversity is germane in that cultural attitudes and beliefs determine how one regards a particular disease–for example, in certain cultures Alzheimer's disease is stigmatized because of its resemblance to mental illness. Attitudes and beliefs impact the concept of caregiving itself and with it the health worker's expectations and practices regarding perceptions of pain, dietary patterns and practices, the use of medications, consultation with physicians, and the level of involvement of family members in the care process. Attitudes towards death and dying vary as well. The patient's cultural background also impacts the above variables, in addition to his/her acceptance of illness and dependency and his/her expectations of care.

While it is difficult to teach about cultural diversity didactically, this important information must be included in the training of all health workers. Additionally, health workers must be encouraged to be sensitive to these important differences in their patients. Assessors must be attuned to the interplay of racial, ethnic, and/or cultural factors in illness and disability and in the patient-family-paid caregiver triad, and must address them in the plan of care. Additionally, the assessor must ascertain that there is adequate communication between the caregiver and care recipient.

At this time, the incorporation of cultural variables into assessment tools is in its infancy, and relevant instruments are not always available. While translation of existing tools into another language is generally preferable to no translation at all, the translated items may be as culturally irrelevant as the questions from which they were originally derived. Thus, caution is advised in the interpretation of findings obtained under these circumstances.

PUTTING IT ALL TOGETHER

The center of the assessment process is the patient and all efforts must be directed at meeting his/her needs, while always considering personhood and dignity.

The goal of assessment is to develop a care plan that will assist the individual in need in an appropriate, efficient and effective way. This plan must be comprehensive yet flexible and must be adaptable to changing needs. Thus, assessment must be ongoing and the more modifications made, the more effective the interventions. Change is not usually indicative of poor planning; but may be an indication of a first-line response to evolving needs. The goal of health providers is to maximize remaining function and reduce dependency when possible.

MEASUREMENT ISSUES REGARDING HOME CARE

There is a paucity of data regarding home care recipients and outcomes of interventions. This information gap is related to major methodological problems in the measurement of aspects of home care. Difficulties include:

1. The *comparability* of patients is difficult to establish because most often there is no single condition involved. Rather, there are frail individuals with several conditions and combinations thereof.
2. There are *ill-defined and multifaceted indications* for home care. Needs are often related to lack of social and/or financial supports rather than severity of illness.
3. *Interrater reliability is uncertain* because of the variability of disciplines and skill levels of assessors.
4. There is *a dearth of premorbid data*, since home care is generally initiated during periods of crisis.
5. There is no *"gold standard" for home care treatment*, and, therefore it is difficult to establish quality assurance criteria. Further, because individual residences are so different to begin with and often very geographically disparate, monitoring is complicated and expensive.
6. Many of the *treated individuals will become sicker*, despite good or excellent care.
7. *Charges may not necessarily represent costs.*
8. Currently used *indicators are "soft,"* e.g., satisfaction or quality of life.

THE FUTURE OF HOME CARE ASSESSMENT

The concept of ADL impairment has been incorporated in proposed health service legislation, and the number of individuals who would be eligible for a given service would depend upon where the cutoff is set (e.g., two impaired ADLs vs. three vs. four) (Kane, Saslow, and Brundage, 1991).

ADL impairment has become a measure of eligibility for nursing home admission and is the basis of the Minimum Data Set (MDS) nursing home assessment tool. This MDS instrument is currently being adapted for use in home care both nationally and internationally (Mor, 1994).

By use of a functional assessment, home care services could be provided on a task basis rather than on a span of time basis. For example, if an individual requires help with bathing and meals, assistance could be provided intermittently during a day only to cover these activities, and one home health aide could perform similar tasks for more than one individual during a given day.

Given an increasing frail elderly and disabled population and limited resources, use of the task-oriented approach might be even more cost-effective when used in a "cluster" or congregate living arrangement. It is, therefore, conceivable that an individual requiring home care in a single-occupant home may have his/her allotted provider time so reduced by travel time that he may not be able to get the needed care at home. Therefore, the task-oriented approach and the underlying assessment have become issues of contention in the litigation currently underway in New York State (Home Care Advisory Committee, Dowd v. Bane, 1993).

CONCLUSION

With the population explosion of the very old, their *extensive* health service needs, and their resounding preference for at-home care, the demand for home health services will increase exponentially. Given the current political climate of shrinking entitlements and other cost-containment strategies, it is likely that home care services will be tightly managed, if not rationed.

Reliable studies are needed to determine the impact of *services/ interventions in much the same way as clinical trials are conducted for pharmaceutical agents*. Qualitative and quantitative impact of home care must be examined in relation to the type of service, intensity, duration and costs. Ideally, a longitudinal study could be devised to follow a cohort of initially well elderly.

All studies will require accurate data collection, based on systematic and comprehensive assessment. This will require valid, and reliable assessment tools and trained assessors to use them. More standardized practices will be required, as will closer monitoring.

Modifications in home care practice will require a different skills mix among those who assess and monitor services and expanded training at every level. With this scenario, costs will likely increase. Thus, to achieve the much desired and sometimes elusive cost-containment, other factors will have to be manipulated, such as the number of individuals eligible and the amount of service to be provided to each. These allocation issues are inextricably bound with the process of assessment. Therefore, it is little wonder that assessment is a topic of keen interest and importance for home health care providers and consumers.

REFERENCES

American Association of Retired Persons. (1994). *Coming up short: Increasing out-of-pocket spending by older Americans.* Washington, D.C.: Public Policy Institute.

Agostinelli, B., Demers, K., Garrigan, D., and Waszynski, C. (1994). "Targeted interventions: Use of the mini-mental state exam," *Journal of Gerontological Nursing*, 20, 15-23.

Applegate, W., Blass, J., and Williams, T.F. (1990). "Instruments for the functional assessment of older patients," *The New England Journal of Medicine*, 322, 1207-1214.

Aronson, M.K. (Ed.). 1994. *Reshaping dementia care: Practice and policy in long term care.* Thousand Oaks, CA: Sage Publications.

Aronson, M.K., Ooi, W.L., Geva, D.L., Masur, D., Blau, A., and Frishman, W. (1991). "Dementia: Age-related incidence, prevalence, and mortality in the old old," *Archives of Internal Medicine*, 151, 989-992.

Beck, A.T. and Beamesderfer, A. (1974). "Assessment of depression: The depression inventory." In Pichot, P. (Ed.), *Psychological measurement in psychopharmacology.* Switzerland: Karger.

Bergner, M., Bobbitt, R.A., Pollard, W.E., and Gilson, B.S. (1976). "Sickness impact profile: Validation of a health status measure," *Medical Care*, 14, 57-67.

Blessed, G., Tomlinson, B.E., and Roth, M. (1968). "The association between quantitative measures of dementia and of senile changes in the cerebral grey matter of elderly subjects," *British Journal of Psychiatry*, 114, 797-811.

Brink, T.L., Yesavage, J.A., Lum, O., Heersema, P.H., Adey, M., and Rose, T.L. (1982). "Screening tests for geriatric depression," *Clinical Gerontologist*, 1, 37-43.

Callahan, D. (1987). *Setting limits: Medical goals in an aging society*. New York, NY: Simon and Schuster.

Cantor, M. (Ed.). (1994). *Family caregiving: Agenda for the future*. San Francisco, CA: American Society on Aging.

Center for the Study of Aging and Human Development, Duke University. (1978). *Multidimensional functional assessment: The OARS methodology*. 2nd Ed. Durham, N.C.: Center for the Study of Aging and Human Development.

Fein, E.B. (July 19, 1994). "Elderly find hardship in haven for young," *The New York Times, Metro*, B1 and B5.

Folstein, M.F., Folstein, S.E., and McHugh, P.R. (1975). "Mini-mental state: A practical method for grading the cognitive state of patients for the clinician," *Journal of Psychiatric Research*, 12, 189-198.

Gurland, B., Kuriansky, J., Sharpe, L., Simon, R., Stiller, P., and Birkett, P. (1977). "The comprehensive assessment and referral evaluation (CARE)–Rationale, development, and reliability: Part II. A factor analysis," *International Journal of Aging and Human Development*, 8, 8-42.

Hamilton, M. (1967). "Development of a rating scale for primary depressive illness," *British Journal of Social Clinical Psychology*, 6, 278-296.

Hollander-Feldman, P., Sapienza, A., and Kane, N. (1990). *Who cares for them? Workers in the home care industry*. Westport, CT: Greenwood Press, Inc.

Home Care Advisory Committee–Dowd v. Bane. (January 12, 1993). *Revise Harri*. New York, NY: Legal Services for the Elderly.

Israel, L., Kozarevic, D., and Sartorius, N. (1984). *Source book of geriatric assessment: Evaluations in gerontology*, Vol. 1, Basel, Switzerland: Karger.

Kane, R. and Kane, R. (1988). *Assessing the elderly: A practical guide to measurement*. Lexington, MA: The Rand Corporation.

Kane, R., Saslow, M., and Brundage, T. (1991). "Using ADL's to establish eligibility for long term care among the cognitively impaired," *The Gerontologist*, 31, 60-66.

Kasper, J. (1988). *Aging alone: Profiles and projections*. New York, NY: Commonwealth Fund Commission on Elderly People Living Alone.

Katz, S., Downs, T.D., Cash, H.R., and Grotz, R.C. (1970). "Progress in the development of the index of ADL," *The Gerontologist*, Part I, 20-30.

Lawton, M.P. (1975). "The Philadelphia Geriatric Center Morale Scale: A Revision," *Journal of Gerontology*, 30, 85-89.

Mahoney, F.I. and Barthel, E.M. (1965). "Functional evaluation: The Barthel index," *Maryland State Medical Journal*, 14, 61-65.

McKegney, P., Aronson, M.K., and Ooi, W.L. (1988). "Identifying depression in the old old: A reliability study," *Psychosomatics*, 29, 175-181.

Milne, J.S., Maule, M.M., Cormack, S., and Williamson, J. (1972). "The design and testing of a questionnaire and examination to assess physical and mental health in older people using a staff nurse as an observer," Journal of Chronic Diseases, 2, 385-405.

Mor, V. (1994). InterRAI client assessment protocols CAPS. Providence, RI: Brown University.

National Association of Professional Geriatric Care Managers. (December 1993). Trends in aging. Tucson, AZ: NAPGCM.

National Health Provider Inventory. (1991). Nursing homes and board and care homes. Hyattsville, MD: NHPI.

Noelker, L. (1994). "The interface between health and social services and family caregivers." In Cantor, M. (Ed.), Family Caregiving: Agenda for the Future. San Francisco, CA: American Society on Aging.

Pearlman, R. (1987). "Development of a functional assessment questionnaire for geriatric patients: The comprehensive older persons' evaluation (COPE)," Journal of Chronic Diseases, 40, 85S-94S.

Pelham, A. and Clark, W. (Eds.). (1986). Managing home care for the elderly: Lessons from community-based agencies. New York, NY: Springer Publishing Company.

Pfeffer, R.I., Kurosaki, T.T., Harrah, C.H., Chance, J.M., and Filos, S. (1982). "Measurement of functional activities in older adults in the community," Journal of Gerontology, 37, 323-329.

Popovich, B., Grubba, C., and Jirovec, M. (1990). "Functional assessments in home care," Home Healthcare Nurse, 8, 16-20.

Reuben, D.B., Wieland, D.L., and Rubenstein, L.Z. (1993). "Functional status assessment of older persons: Concepts and implications," Facts and Research in Gerontology, 12, 63-70.

Schoening, H.A. and Iversen, I.A. (1968). "Numerical scoring of self-care status: A study of the Kenny self-care evaluation," Archives of Physical Medicine and Rehabilitation, 49, 221-229.

United States Department of Health and Human Services. (1990). Healthy People 2000. National Health Promotion and Disease Prevention Objectives, DHHS Publication #(PHS) 91-50212. Washington, DC: U.S. Government Printing Office.

Zung, W.W.K. (1965). "A self rating depression scale," Archives of General Psychiatry, 12, 63-70.

Chapter 11

Case Management in Home and Community Care

Joan Quinn, RN, MSN

As the paradigm shifts from institutional care to home care without significant government sponsored health care reform, it is an important time to look at all systems of care in the community setting. The community care system, because of very limited public or private financial support, has not developed in the same way as institutional care. Therefore, community care may be more fragmented and difficult to access, especially by older adults with chronic long-term care needs.

Even so, the primary focus for care has moved from the institutional setting to a continuum of care in the community. It has moved from a specialty care focus to a primary care base; from treating illness to maintaining wellness; from caring for individuals to improving health status for populations; from managing departments to managing a process; and from being an individual provider to being a partner in a care continuum.

These changes are evident in the rapid development of managed care entities such as health maintenance organizations, physician-hospital managed care programs and the formation of joint ventures which are attempting to integrate acute and long-term care systems.

[Haworth co-indexing entry note]: "Case Management in Home and Community Care." Quinn, Joan. Co-published simultaneously in *Journal of Gerontological Social Work* (The Haworth Press, Inc.) Vol. 24, No. 3/4, 1995, pp. 233-248; and: *New Developments in Home Care Services for the Elderly: Innovations in Policy, Program, and Practice* (ed: Lenard W. Kaye) The Haworth Press, Inc., 1995, pp. 233-248. Single or multiple copies of this article are available from The Haworth Document Delivery Service [1-800-342-9678, 9:00 a.m. - 5:00 p.m. (EST)].

© 1995 by The Haworth Press, Inc. All rights reserved.

These models all emphasize less care rather than more and attempt to educate plan enrollees about disease prevention through programs such as the negative effects of smoking, good dietary habits and the value of exercise in maintaining health (Swanson, 1993). These dramatic shifts have resulted in a very unstable acute medical care system in which home and community-based care and case management will achieve new importance, emphasis, and use.

For a long time, parallel health and social systems in the United States have been developing which have not been beneficial to their users for a number of reasons, including eligibility requirements with regard to income, entry to the program based on functional disability, and/or specific categorical disease diagnoses. In most instances, program entry variables are dissimilar in focus. For example, in order to enter a program funded by Medicaid, one must be poor and fragile physically while Medicare entry criteria include age and acute illness. The health and social systems have become more complex as they have evolved and multiplied and have caused users of care to be confused about how to access, use, and pay for services that these systems deliver. The situation has become even more confusing for older persons with multiple complex diagnoses and functional disabilities who may meet some but not all criteria in each program.

IMPORTANCE OF A CONTINUUM OF CARE

The value of a continuum of care for individuals has evolved over time. Why a continuum of care? First, it is felt that health care costs, whether community-based or institutional, may be decreased because of more appropriate care being delivered to consumers in a nonduplicative service system response to their particular needs. This belief is especially valid for those receiving multiple medical and social support services in the home care setting. Second is the dramatic population shift from a young society to an old-old society, where increasingly significant numbers of older adults are living well into their 80s and beyond, when they are more apt to need multiple services. These very old adults often are living in the community with and without formal assistance. Their family caregivers can easily be in their 60s and experiencing their own physical problems, which complicates their caregiving responsibilities to their 85-year-old mother or father. In some instances, it is not unusual to have the reverse situation, the 85 year old caring for the 60 year old. The extent to which the older caregiver can sustain the caregiving is difficult at best.

DEVELOPMENT OF HOME HEALTH CARE

Home and community-based care is not a new phenomenon. When England enacted its first formal social welfare legislation in 1601, it contained a home care provision (Applebaum and Austin, 1990). Within the last 30 years such care has expanded greatly, fueled by growth in the number of elderly; the rising cost of nursing home care; and the availability of federal funding sources such as Medicare, Medicaid, and Title III of the Older Americans Act. Medicare funds are earmarked for acute care prescribed by a physician with the expectation that the individual will be rehabilitated within a short period. Medicaid funds pay for both acute and long-term care when certain eligibility criteria are met, namely income and medical necessity.

In 1993, data from a national home and hospice survey published by the Department of Health and Human Services reported that people over age 65 comprise 74.5% of those receiving home health care, and 71.5% of these were receiving home hospice care. Of the people over age 65, 18.7% were over age 85; 16% were between age 80 and 81; and 15.7% were between ages 75 and 79. Of the 1.5 million people receiving home care in 1992, 1.1 million were elderly. Such staggering figures create both challenges and opportunities for home care providers and case management organizations and individuals (National Association for Home Care, 1993).

EVOLUTION OF LONG-TERM CARE
CASE MANAGEMENT

In the 1970s, concurrent with the growth of home and community-based long-term care, the Department of Health and Human

Services funded national research and demonstration projects which created a case management service that integrated the health and social support systems of care for the consumer, thus improving access to care, creating new alternatives and overseeing the affordability and delivery of service as well as its quality. There was a redefinition of health and social support services for the consumer served by the case management program which was more responsive to their needs and which provided care options for them in a more integrated system of short- and long-term care. Although case management provided integration for clients, the traditional system of care did not change. People not eligible for case management still struggled with health and social services and their financing systems, usually during a time of crisis.

More recently, states have developed care management programs for targeted frail individuals needing formal long-term care service in the community and institutions, using and adopting components of these early state research and demonstration programs. Most of these programs are funded under a combination of Medicaid waiver and state funds.

Further, new long-term care insurance products, especially the Partnership programs now available in several states, include a case management benefit to facilitate access to and control of long-term care services to policyholders. OBRA 1990 recognized nonprovider case management as an optional Medicaid service. The 1992 reauthorization of the Older Americans Act specified that independent case management was a service eligible for funding. With the aging of America, the age 85+ segment of American citizens is the fastest growing group and also the group most likely to need long-term care services. Long-term care case management promises to become even more important for the 85+ segment of the elderly population.

OBJECTIVES OF LONG-TERM CARE CASE MANAGEMENT

Long-term care case management for frail older and/or disabled populations has numerous objectives. Some are primarily client-oriented while others are system-oriented (Applebaum and Austin, 1990).

Client-Oriented Objectives

- *To assure that services given are appropriate to client needs.* Development of care plans by case managers rather than service providers will help assure that service prescriptions meet multiple client needs; include both formal and informal services and change as needed. In contrast, care plans developed by service providers tend to include only their own offerings.
- *To monitor appropriateness of long-term care services.* Monitoring ensures that services are provided as scheduled and satisfactorily. It also allows for a quick response to changes in the client's needs and to prevent further deterioration in the client's condition. For example, if the client becomes forgetful about taking medications, the case manager will set up a way to assure medication compliance.
- *To improve client access to the continuum of long-term care services.* A client seeking services may have difficulty obtaining them because of agency regulations, long waiting lists, and the need to select from multiple providers. A case manager should simplify this by being the point of entry and primary contact for clients.
- *To support the client's caregivers.* Case management will see that a client's informal supporters have respite from the responsibilities of caregiving when needed.
- *To serve as a bridge between institutional and community-based care systems.* When case managers follow their clients as they enter and leave hospitals and nursing homes, they can facilitate their return to the community by coordinating the formal and informal services that will make this possible.

System-Oriented Objectives

- *To facilitate the development of noninstitutional services.* Because care planning involves service prescriptions, case managers are in a position to promote the development of new services and reduce service duplications within a community.
- *To promote quality in long-term care service delivery.* Because they monitor the services their clients receive, case managers

can influence their quality. Quality service also includes the case management service.

- *To enhance the coordination of long-term care service delivery.* If clients are receiving services from multiple providers, care managers will assure that the services are properly sequenced and scheduled.
- *To target individuals most at-risk of nursing home placement in order to prevent inappropriate institutionalization.* Case management, in conjunction with adequate community-based long-term care services, can prevent premature institutionalization. Through preadmission screening, case management can often divert individuals to community-based services.
- *To contain cost by controlling client access to services.* If case managers serve as the initial screen for access to services, they can help contain long-term care costs. Each case management function supports the goal of assuring services are based on need and appropriately used.

ADMINISTRATION OF CASE MANAGEMENT SERVICES

Case management services are administered by numerous modalities. These include:

- Municipal agencies;
- Private, nonprofit agencies;
- Individual geriatric case managers;
- Community service providers;
- Proprietary agencies.

Most case management programs funded with state and federal monies have not been administered by agencies which also provide services. Rather, publicly-funded case management agencies contract with home health and social service agencies for services for their clients (Quinn, 1993), who often have multiple, complex, chronic health, social, and/or cognitive problems. The services provided have included living options, financial counseling, legal advice, home health services (nursing, physical, occupational, and speech therapy), and social support services (homemaker, companion, home-delivered meals, adult day care, emergency response systems).

Case management organizations typically employ either an individual or team approach in their practices. The advantage of the former approach is that clients have a single contact; the main disadvantage is that it is professionally isolating and does not allow for easy collaboration with peers. In the latter approach, social service personnel and nurses work together to solve problems. Also, team members can readily substitute for one another which provides continuity of service to clients and helps minimize case manager burnout.

CASE MANAGER QUALIFICATIONS

In most publicly-funded case management organizations, case managers are registered nurses or social workers. Geriatric case managers in private practice may have human services or gerontology degrees as well as nursing or social work degrees.

The National Council on Aging's care management standards, established by its National Institute on Community-Based Long-Term Care, define case manager professional qualifications as follows:

- Graduate of an accredited four-year college or university with a degree in nursing, social service, gerontology, health or related field and at least two years experience in a human service field; or
- Graduate of a master's level professional program with a degree in social work or nursing and one year experience in a human service field.

Even with these credentials, new case managers require extensive orientation before they are able to carry a full case load. In addition to mastering the functions of case management, they must handle the stress of dealing with a frail client population. Also the demands of community-based rather than institutional care are a challenge. In addition to clinical skills, the case manager must acquire knowledge about available health, social service, and financial resources.

Relationships with clients being served at home also differ from relationships with institutionalized clients (Quinn, 1993). Case managers must always keep in mind that clients have the authority to control and decide what services are to be provided. They must think of themselves as invited guests and be sensitive to their clients' wishes.

CASELOAD SIZE

If the client mix includes primarily very frail people with numerous needs, a case manager cannot successfully manage many clients. Another determinant is the size of the geographic area covered by the agency. Having a case manager assistant who can help with day-to-day client management allows for a larger caseload size. Availability of long-term care services and support for case management within the community also influence caseload size (Applebaum and Austin, 1990).

In long-term care demonstration projects caseload varied as follows:

Project	Average caseload
Pentastar (Florida)	35 - 40
Long-Term Care Project (San Diego)	37 - 46
MSSP (California)	50 - 67
TRIAGE, Inc.	60 - 70
Community Long-Term Care Project (South Carolina)	75 - 85

As caseload size increases, case managers typically say they have less time to spend on such case management activities as monitoring and reassessment (Applebaum and Austin, 1990). Some may even question whether they are providing case management in certain instances.

CASE MANAGEMENT FUNCTIONS

Within the profession, six functions are generally considered to be "core" or essential functions.

Comprehensive Assessment

Case management begins with a comprehensive client assessment. This function or service is the foundation for appropriate long-term care.

Comprehensive assessment typically involves a face-to-face interview between the client and case manager at the client's home. During this meeting, which generally lasts two or three hours, the case manager collects information about the client, using a standardized assessment instrument or form. Data are collected about the client's health, emotional/behavioral status, functional capacity, cognitive capacity, support system (family, friends, neighbors), environment, and financial status. Case managers use this information to determine the client's needs for services and whether supports and resources are available which will enable the individual to remain at home.

Care Plan Development

The comprehensive assessment is the foundation for another "core" case management function, care plan development. Schneider (1988) says care planning:

- involves the client and caregivers in the process;
- is problem-oriented and goal directed;
- makes plans for a specific period of time;
- involves both formal and informal services;
- is cost conscious;
- results in a written document.

Perhaps the most important aspect of care plan development to remember is that care plan decisions ultimately rest with the client. Decisions which differ from the case manager's ideas of appropriate care should not be a measure of the case manager's success or failure in care planning (Quinn, 1993).

Care Plan Implementation

Care plan implementation is the process of putting the care plan into action in a timely and cost-effective manner. It involves knowledge of community resources and available funding sources; negotiating with formal and informal providers of care; and teaching clients and caregivers to use needed social and health services. In many instances, implementation involves actual purchase of services. It also requires that care managers take consumer preferences into account, including their cultural beliefs and language.

Monitoring

After a care plan is in place, care managers need to monitor its effectiveness. Monitoring enables the care manager to evaluate the consumer's condition. Has it improved, remained the same, or declined? It also assesses the adequacy of the care plan. Is the consumer receiving the services needed to maintain maximum independence? A third purpose is to evaluate the services provided. Are the paid services appropriate, cost-effective, of high quality, and delivered as planned? Are the informal service providers meeting their obligations? Are the informal caregivers coping with the client situation? Finally, monitoring enables the care manager to make adjustments as necessary.

Monitoring includes phone or face-to-face contact with consumers; verbal or written reports from service providers; and consumer or family-initiated contacts with the case manager to report changes in consumer status or in the quality of services delivered.

Reassessment

Reassessments determine a consumer's continued need for services, including case management. They may be as time-consuming as the original assessment and should include collection of abbreviated similar data. Reassessments ensure the successful targeting of resources. They also enable the care manager to evaluate care plan appropriateness and reestablish a personal relationship with the client.

In doing reassessments, care managers need to know how to measure goal achievement and progress towards goals; how to conduct a reassessment without assuming the client's status has not changed; how to adjust care plans; and how to help the client adjust to changes caused by the reassessment.

Publicly-funded case management services often require reassessments at stated intervals. In other cases, reassessments occur when there is a noticeable change in the client's condition. There tends to be some variation in the quality of reassessments. Case managers with a large number of clients may have a tendency to shortcut this process. Also, many case managers feel they know their clients well and don't need to complete a comprehensive reassessment. Some clients also question the need to undergo a comprehensive reassessment.

Termination and Discharge

Discharge (also called termination or case closure) from case management services occurs when the case manager no longer provides case management services. Discharge occurs when the consumer no longer wishes case management services; becomes ineligible for services; or exhausts benefits. Discharge also occurs when consumers remain stable for a long period. This allows scarce case management services to be used appropriately.

Ideally, payer requirements would permit consumers to continue to receive long-term care services even though they no longer wish or need case management services. In such situations, consumers would be discharged from case management but would not end all formal ties with case management.

Candidates for discharge include consumers who can learn to manage their care providers (self-directed care); consumers whose families can assume case management responsibilities; and mentally competent consumers who have reliable caregiver support and are receiving services from a single high quality provider.

STAFFING A CASE MANAGEMENT AGENCY

Individuals receiving the benefits of case management and residing in communities are similar to the rest of the population in ethnicity, diversity, and cultural roots. Case management agencies should, therefore, strive to assemble staffs with backgrounds similar to the population they serve. When this happens, rapport between case manager and client will usually be more easily achieved.

Case management agencies must also seek individuals who have or can develop certain skills. First, case managers must be *knowledgeable about the agency's target population*. They need familiarity with the aging process, cultural roots of the population, and how long-term disability affects behavior.

Second, case managers need to have *effective interpersonal skills*. They must always treat clients with respect and be sensitive to their needs. They must be able to advocate for their clients with service providers, physicians, and community agencies.

Third, case managers must have *good interviewing skills*. These include listening carefully and asking additional questions to validate information. During an assessment, observation of clients and how they function in their surroundings also provides invaluable information.

Fourth, case managers must be *knowledgeable about community programs and agencies*. They must be familiar with eligibility criteria for local, state, and federal programs and the cost of various services. They must be able to help clients apply to the programs and to negotiate for the services the client needs.

Fifth, case managers must have good *telephone communication skills*. Most case manager contact with provider agencies is by telephone. They need to be sensitive to provider concerns while arranging for services, monitoring service delivery, or handling a crisis.

Sixth, case managers need good *time management skills*. Each day case managers face numerous tasks, including client admissions, clients in crisis, documentation, staff meetings, routine client follow-up, meetings with provider agencies, supervisory/peer consultations, etc.

PRIVATE GERIATRIC CARE MANAGEMENT vs. PUBLICLY-FUNDED AND NOT-FOR-PROFIT CARE MANAGEMENT

Within the last five years, private geriatric care management has grown rapidly. Many factors are responsible for this trend (Kaye, 1992). In the first place, the number of older persons is growing rapidly. More than one in 10 Americans is now over age 65 (Kasper, 1988). By the year 2030, about 21% of the population will be age 65 or older.

A second factor is the economic status of the older population. The 65+ age group is more affluent than all age groups under age 45.

A third factor is the increasing complexity and difficulty in maneuvering within the network of gerontological services. It is almost impossible for a lay person to locate the services needed without help.

Yet another factor is the growing difficulty of families to provide ongoing care for their elders. The two-income family is becoming the norm, and many families are widely dispersed geographically, which further limits their ability to provide care.

The resistance of many older adults to seek help from public programs as well as the short life span, inadequate funding, and uneven quality of services available in many communities also has contributed to the growth of private care management.

Finally, health and social services professionals are recognizing that private practice gives them more personal satisfaction, higher incomes, and increased status than may be found in publicly-funded care management.

Private geriatric care managers have their own national organization, the National Association of Professional Geriatric Care Managers. Founded in 1982, it is growing rapidly. Between 1990 and 1992, for example, membership doubled. Future growth seems assured since not-for-profit case managers can now also join as fully participating members (Cress, 1992).

For-profit and not-for-profit case management have more similarities than differences. Both types of case managers perform the same core functions; help families solve long-term care problems; and must be knowledgeable about reimbursement and community-based services. Also, both know that they need to educate the public about case management and that their activities must include network building and interdisciplinary coordination with other health care professionals.

Both for-profit and not-for-profit case managers recognize the need for high practice standards within the profession. The National Association of Professional Geriatric Care Managers and the Case Management Institute of Connecticut Community Care, Inc., a private, nonprofit organization which is a pioneer and pacesetter in long-term care case management, have teamed up to establish the National Academy of Certified Care Managers (NACCM). Its purpose is to advance the quality of care management services; assure competence to perform care management; create validated, standardized examinations; and test skills, knowledge and practice ethics. The organization is developing a care management credential and the first test administration for that credential is scheduled for December 1995.

Many for-profit case management organizations are based on not-for-profit models. However, they tend to be quite small; 65% have one or two case managers on staff and 17% have three or four case managers. Their services are not generally reimbursable through Medicare, Medicaid, or private insurance. Clients or their family members typically pay case management fees.

QUALITY IMPROVEMENT IN CASE MANAGEMENT

As in many other endeavors, quality improvement is an essential aspect of long-term care case management (Geron and Chassler, 1994). It not only protects consumers but also enhances case management clinical practice.

What constitutes a quality improvement system? In the first place, it should clearly state what constitutes quality community-based as well as institutional care and case management practice.

Second, all staff members of a case management organization or practice should be aware of quality goals and expectations. Training activities, audits, policies and protocols should all reflect quality goals.

Third, a quality improvement program should empower consumers to have a stake in the quality of services they receive by encouraging them to make choices about their care, educating them about their rights, establishing procedures to make complaints about services and to notify case managers of problems.

Fourth, a quality improvement system should include a Consumer Bill of Rights and Responsibilities. Among its provisions: responsibility of case management to payers and management of potential conflicts of interest.

Fifth, procedures should be in place that motivate case managers to improve the quality of the services they provide and permit assessment of case manager clinical skills and competencies in carrying out the core case management functions.

Sixth, a quality improvement system should regularly gather information from consumers about their satisfaction with case management and formal in-home services.

Seventh, the system should include corrective strategies for identified quality problems in case management or provider services.

MECHANISMS FOR EVALUATING
CASE MANAGEMENT SERVICE

As the paradigm for care continues to shift away from institutions toward home and community, case management will increasingly be key to bridging the acute, sub-acute and community care systems and to meeting consumer needs. To demonstrate the value of case management, mechanisms are evolving to measure its success. Many organizations survey consumers to find out whether case management and the services provided met their expectations. At Connecticut Community Care, Inc., for example, we interview 50 randomly selected consumers by phone each quarter. Cost-effectiveness is another way to measure the value of case management. This is especially important for publicly-funded programs. They carefully examine whether case management has resulted in lower expenditures of public monies than would have occurred without this service. Feedback from family and other informal caregivers is a third way to measure the value of case management. Has it given them the necessary respite to enable them to continue to fulfill their very important caregiving role?

REFERENCES

Applebaum, R. and Austin, C. (1990). *Long-Term Care Case Management.* New York, NY: Springer Publishing Company.

Cress, C. (1992). "The Business of For-Profit Case Management," *Journal of Case Management,* 1, 113-116.

Geron, S. M. and Chassler, D. (1994). *Guidelines for Case Management Practice Across the Long-Term Care Continuum.* Bristol, CT: Connecticut Community Care, Inc.

Kasper, J. D. (1988). *Aging Alone: Profiles and Projections.* New York, NY: The Commonwealth Fund Commission on Elderly People Living Alone.

Kaye, L. (1992). "The Evolution of Private Geriatric Care Management," *Journal of Case Management,* 1, 103-107.

National Association for Home Care. (1993). Report No. 526, August 20.

Quinn, J. (1993). *Successful Case Management in Long-Term Care.* New York, NY: Springer Publishing Company.

Schneider, B. (1988). "Care Planning: The Core of Case Management," *Generations,* 12, No. 5, 16-18.

Swanson, K. H. (1993). "Nursing as Informed Caring for the Well-Being of Others," *Image,* 25, 352-357.

PART IV:
INNOVATION FROM ABROAD

Chapter 12

Trends and Developments in Home Care Services: An International Perspective

Abraham Monk, PhD
Carole Cox, DSW

The last two decades witnessed the upsurge of a generalized commitment to community care for the frail aged in most of the developed countries of the world. The reasons for this turn in public policy toward home care services, as opposed to the previous institutionalization trend, are epitomized by two widely held ideological positions that were formulated in western Europe. One underscores cost efficiency and cost saving criteria. The other is centered around quality of life concerns.

The best known expression of the first argument is contained in the policy of "substitution" of services adopted by the government of the Netherlands. It defines substitution as the systematic replacement of costly services with less expensive ones, provided the latter adequately meet the extent of felt need. This policy implies not only the adoption of home care as the alternative for institutional services but also the sponsorship of informal supports as preferable to formal, community organized services. The policy in reference is

[Haworth co-indexing entry note]: "Trends and Developments in Home Care Services: An International Perspective." Monk, Abraham, and Carole Cox. Co-published simultaneously in *Journal of Gerontological Social Work* (The Haworth Press, Inc.) Vol. 24, No. 3/4, 1995, pp. 251-270; and: *New Developments in Home Care Services for the Elderly: Innovations in Policy, Program, and Practice* (ed: Lenard W. Kaye) The Haworth Press, Inc., 1995, pp. 251-270. Single or multiple copies of this article are available from The Haworth Document Delivery Service [1-800-342-9678, 9:00 a.m. - 5:00 p.m. (EST)].

© 1995 by The Haworth Press, Inc. All rights reserved.

predicated upon a hypothetical future "shrinkage" scenario, which assumes that self-care and primary prevention will become generalized behaviors, and that this trend will ultimately result in improved health status and a lower need for services among the aged (Kastelein, Dijkstra and Schouten, 1989).

The prospects of a service "shrinkage" have been similarly anticipated for the United States, based however on a possible "backlash" trend among young adult cohorts. Binstock (1983) has thus suggested that taxpayers under the age of 65 may refuse to continue footing an increasingly larger services bill for a steadily growing and progressively older senior population. In other words, as the number of aged persons increases, services may become less readily available for all of them. Social planners and policy makers will have to find ways of doing more with less. The renewed appeals to filial responsibility and family caregiving, the weakening of universal entitlement provisions in aging-related policies, the tightening of eligibility rules and the virtual placement of expenditure ceilings in many service programs in the United States point, indeed, to cost containment strategies in the face of projections of greater need.

The second argument is contained in the principle of "normalization" spelled out in the Swedish Social Services Act of 1982 and the subsequent Health and Medical Services Act of 1983 which declared, among others, that individuals should be assisted to live and function in their own homes, so that they may continue leading their habitual independent existence. The Dutch government also came out with a comprehensive policy statement that similarly included an "integration" objective. This aspiration actually transcends the provision of community care as it also advocates facilitating the social participation of the aged in all spheres of life and as part of their natural communities of residence (Ministry of Welfare, Health and Cultural Affairs, 1991). Looming beneath these policy goals is the inexorable demographic imperative of a relentless process of population aging. In the case of the Netherlands, the percentage of people over the age of 65 will almost double from its 1980 level of 11.5 to 21.2 percent by 2030 (Kastelein et al., 1989).

THE QUEST FOR NORMALIZATION

Although a praiseworthy aspiration, normalization has proven difficult to attain and even more to hold on to it. Analyzing service utilization data from 24 Swedish counties, Berg et al. (1988) observed that during the 1965 to 1975 decade nursing home beds continued growing but at a modest 17 percent pace while the number of home care recipients expanded by 73 percent. However, both institutional and home care services declined at almost identical rates–13 and 16 percent–respectively, in the course of the following decade. Thorslund (1992) similarly notes that although the number of persons in Sweden receiving home care services more than tripled during the twenty year period that started in the early 1960s, the capacity of this service system peaked and actually had begun to decline in the mid 1980s. It simply could not keep up with the costs of a seemingly bottomless demand level. Initial euphoria faded and it now appears that home care can no longer compensate for the previous deliberate containment of the rate of institutional placements. The ultimate albeit unintended consequence of "normalization" is that both the institutional and the noninstitutional services have been beating, in effect, a retreat. This would not be immediately apparent from the volume of home care hours of service which actually tripled from a total of 35 million in 1965 to 105 million in 1990. Not all these, however, were allocated to direct service or client contact, as the proportion of time consumed by case conferences, consultation, training, travel, paper work and bureaucratic chores has, in fact, grown at a greater pace (Szebehely and Eliasson, 1991). It would appear then that their overhead or indirect costs are growing voraciously, to the obvious detriment of the direct provision of services. Moreover, the percentage of elderly 65 years of age and older who received formal care–either home help or institutional care–declined by 29 percent between 1980 and 1991 (Szebehely, 1993), and the trend seems to accelerate. In 1992 alone the proportion of those 80+ receiving home care services fell an additional 10 percent, from a 40 percent level in 1991 to 36 percent (Statistics Sweden, 1993).

If normalization is associated with a virtual decline in the provision of formal services, who fills the gap? It is easy to guess: the informal system, that is, the relatives. These are, for the most part, daughters between the ages of 50 and 65, most of whom are gainfully employed and do not reside with the care recipient. The proportion of elderly who depend upon the help of a nonresiding relative has increased by 44 percent in Sweden, between 1980 and 1989 (Szebehely, 1993).

THE QUEST FOR "SUBSTITUTION"

"Substitution" may not have fared better than "normalization." To begin with there was initial evidence, in the case of the Netherlands, that although home help services can partially substitute for "Old People's Homes," the cost of home care ended up exceeding that of the institutional facilities, once home care services are required for more than 8 hours of assistance per week (Goewie, 1988). The assumption that home care is economically more advantageous than institutional care, and consequently a desirable substitute, has not been found to be true by Guillemard and Frossard (1993) when comparing the costs of living at home with those of an institution in a sample of persons 75 years of age and older in the French departments of Doubs and Loire-Atlantique. In a similar vein, and when reviewing a series of field studies conducted in Amsterdam, Breda and the province of Groningen, Pijl (1991) initially warns that it is impossible to compare costs between intensive home care and "intramural" (hospital and/or nursing home) care because reliable information about the latter was not yet available. Further on the author raises doubts whether a significant financial difference will be found altogether. In any event, the Social and Cultural Planning Council of the Netherlands projected that substitution policies would lead to a reduction ranging from 5 to 15 percent in service expenditures, a claim some analysts find too optimistic and even if correct, too modest to compensate for the increase in service demand.

THE SPONSORSHIP
OF SYSTEMATIC EXPERIMENTATION

Policymakers remain committed to pursue the implementation of the two goals in reference–normalization and substitution–even if the initial results have been rather modest or ambiguous. There is no turning back to square one.

A positive effect of that implementation quest, at least in Western Europe, has been the extensive and systematic volume of experimentation with new patterns and methodologies of service delivery. Once home care services were accorded a higher policy and budgetary priority, several national governments launched a series of demonstrations largely aimed to test whether these services do in effect what they are supposed to do; that is, neutralize the risk of institutionalization and then, whether they constitute in effect an efficient "substitute" for the more costly levels of institutional care.

Innovative projects tend to include an assortment of types or modalities of service. The most common are:

1. Development of new diagnostic methods aimed at better targeting and prioritizing the provision of services.
2. Coordination of the different subcomponents of the home care service system.
3. Coordination of home care with housing on one hand, and health care services on the other.
4. Gap filling community-based services such as day care and respite care.
5. Recruitment, training, retention and skills updating of professional and paraprofessional personnel cadres.
6. Procurement of new funding sources to cover cost increments.
7. Simplification of budgetary allocation and service reimbursement procedures.
8. User-friendly communication technology for monitoring and quick response in emergency situations.
9. Prosthetic devices that facilitate mobility and functional independent capacity.
10. Incentives for consumer and community participation in the planning, organization and operation of home-delivered services.
11. Institution of recourse, appeal and redress procedures for cases of consumer dissatisfaction.
12. Integration of formal and informal services.

13. Administrative and operational mechanisms for flexible, easy and multidirectional transition from service to service within the long-term care continuum.

It is rather difficult to keep a systematic inventory of all innovations in any given national society. Some innovations are specifically instituted by legislative mandate and are usually national in scope. They consequently require formal sanction and explicitly set uniform guidelines for their implementation and evaluation. These service experiments are relatively easy to monitor. This is not the case with innovations that spring up spontaneously at the local level because they often go unrecorded. Only those initiatives that prove to be successful or popular are disseminated by word of mouth, throughout the service network until the media and public authorities take notice. However, it is not easy for grass roots departures to prosper and remain sustained unless tolerated and even favored by local decision makers and public authorities. Once the latter perceive the potential political or programmatic utility of these novel treatment approaches they may well adopt them as their own. The apparent gap between the formal and the spontaneous innovations is thus narrowed.

Baldock and Evers (1991) affirm that innovations, far from being neutral are actually embedded in the "care culture" of each country. The new service modalities conceived and tested by each society consequently reflect its traditions, dominant interests, funding capacity and philosophies of service. It may well appear that certain categories of innovations are particularly underscored in a given country–the United Kingdom, for instance, giving more attention to the linkage between the formal and the informal or volunteer services sectors–but, as is the case with most Western European countries, they all tend to be committed to a certain degree of pluralism or mixed strategy. While some governments seem to be more committed to finding empirical validation for some of their innovative ideas, no country appears to have an exclusive hold on a single category of experimentation.

The principle of "substitution" is a case in point. Several countries have embarked in testing its hypothesized merits from the perspective of one or more of the above categories. The Nether-

lands stands out, however, for its rather comprehensive and systematic program of experimentation conducted between 1988 and
1991. These interventions tend to cluster around three main foci
that overlap and combine most of the experimental categories listed
above:

1. New patterns of budgetary allocations, including personal
   budgets for care and cash allowances.
2. Flexible uses of sheltered or congregate housing.
3. Decentralization of planning implementation of long-term
   care services at the local level, with more intensive use of case
   management methods.

DIRECT CASH PAYMENTS TO CARE RECIPIENTS

The use of care allowances for relatives or friends who provide
regular care have been common in Great Britain and the Scandina-
vian countries. The Invalid Care allowance was introduced in England as early as 1976 and seems to be the way of the future today,
as 59 countries have already been offering direct cash grants since
1981, according to a survey conducted by the United Seniors Health
Cooperative (*Productive Aging News*, 1994). Moreover, a similar
idea has been introduced in the original Clinton plan for long-term
care services, as a substitute or an alternative to the current vendor
payments system under both Medicare and Medicaid.

A related strategy, that of recruiting relatives as paid home care
providers, has been extensively utilized in Norway, given the high
turnover rates of home care workers. Policymakers in that country
observed that little can be done to reverse the unskilled and lower
status of home care personnel and that consequently it is not worth-
while investing too much in their training. The advantages of paying relatives are their obvious greater sense of commitment and the
possibility that they may be willing to take on more than just their
frail relative and extend their attention to other persons in need in
the immediate vicinity.

Some countries have instituted direct cash payments as a restrictive rather than a generalized policy. Israel, for instance, began
offering cash payments in 1986 to eligible elderly assessed as re-

quiring assistance in order to remain in their homes. However, these cash benefits are allocated only to persons living with a relative who provides care and in those instances where services are not available in the community. Cash is not given to those living alone; these elderly must receive services. Thus, although cash benefits are available, the emphasis remains on services.

Recent legislation in Germany gives recipients the choice between home care services and a cash allowance. If they opt for the latter, the funds must be exclusively used to obtain services from their immediate informal networks, neighbors included. These caregivers, in turn, will also be earning pension credits for the time spent taking care of their dependent older relatives. Policies authorizing direct payments to patients are generally based on two debatable assumptions:

1. That the recipient has access to a roster of home care providers, and is then able to make an informed decision. Regrettably the "products" in question, that is, the service agencies, are not being displayed for public scrutiny as goods on supermarket shelves. Frail and disabled consumers rarely have a chance to shop around, and even when they or their caregivers obtain detailed information about their choice of provider, they usually do not know the workers that will be assigned to assist them.

2. That putting cash in the hands of the consumers empowers them to bargain and negotiate. In other words, it gives them the leverage to award or withdraw the job assignment. This is a logical but highly implausible premise in a sellers market. In most countries the home care agencies are overburdened, as the demand for services exceeds the supply. Applicants for services may then be deferred, placed on waiting lists or shifted to other services. Consumers do not have much to choose from and end up taking whatever they can get.

Cash payments are meaningless unless there is an adequate supply of services to purchase from and, as is often the case, needed services tend to be in short supply in small cities and sparsely populated areas. It then becomes a matter of debate as to whether a government is abrogating its responsibilities by not initiating the provision of services needed by a substantial population group (Evers and Leichsenring, 1994).

The individual care subsidy demonstration in Rotterdam was launched in 1988 with the intent to overcome some of those service deficiencies. The objective was to enable frail older persons to continue living in their homes as long as possible, by means of both an individual care subsidy and a "care mediator." These mediators were professionals who had the authority to apply the care subsidies to the purchase of services, in order to supplement or fill gaps left by the more traditional home care services.

Each individual budget had assigned a maximum subsidy of about one-fourth of the equivalent average cost of institutional care. The 75 elderly that participated in this demonstration were taken from waiting lists for residential homes and were matched with a control group which did not receive any of the services. At the end of the three year period, 38% of those in the experiment moved to a nursing home as compared to 73% in the control group. It is also important to note that although the level of disability between the two groups was comparable at the onset of the experiment, by the third interview, those in the control group exhibited a significantly higher level of impairments.

Care mediators did not have the authority to command services and were dependent upon the good will of the independent providers. These agencies were truly forthcoming with their cooperation but the evaluators wondered whether this positive response had to do with the fact that they were dealing with a time-limited demonstration project rather than a more permanent policy requirement (Coolen, 1993).

SHELTERED HOUSING

"Sheltered" houses in the Netherlands largely correspond to the American congregate care model and to the Swedish "service" houses. They consist of services–enriched forms of independent living, usually in an apartment complex, which includes an electronic alarm system linked to a nearby service center, long-term care facility or even a hospital. Sheltered houses could thus constitute networks of community residential satellites affiliated with a central service station for health emergency purposes. However, no two sheltered housing complexes are alike. The model resists standardization because one of its main objectives is, precisely, to foster grass roots self-determination.

The Gooyer House of Amsterdam is an appropriate example. Its multistoried building is situated on a busy corner, just across from an open street market and residents are found to watch street activity from their windows or to go out to mingle with the daily shoppers. They enjoy the daily hustle and bustle of their immediate community and on frequent occasions they may bump into old neighbors and acquaintances. They are well-known to the stand owners, from whom they buy their daily fresh produce.

The building is part of an entire block of apartment houses, lacking any distinguishing institutional features. Moreover, all buildings converge into and share an inner court, which includes a childrens' playground and a small landscaped garden. The Gooyer House residents frequently sit in the court and socialize with tenants of all ages, including children and some of their own relatives who happen to live in those adjacent buildings.

Residents occupy their own studio type units in a cluster of about four to six apartments with a common social and recreational space. A cluster contains residents of different levels of disability in the expectation that they will help each other and share their skills. Relatives and friends come at all hours, especially after work, to also lend a hand. The central administration monitors the independent viability of each of those clusters and, depending on circumstances such as infirmities, hospitalizations, or the aggravation of a condition, will determine whether additional home help inputs or supportive services are required on a temporary or continuous basis. In all instances, the sheltered house aims to preserve the active participation of the informal system in the daily chores as well as their individual integration in the surrounding environment. In the specific case of Gooyer, the residents obtained a liquor license and operate a pub and cafeteria on the ground floor open to the public. The profits from these operations are applied to the costs of running and improving the facility.

Two other Dutch experiments conducted in the late 1980s attempted to blend congregate–or sheltered–housing with institution-type services. The intent was to ascertain whether such a combination would lead to: (1) a more parsimonious use of formal services;

(2) a more intensive use of informal services than in traditional nursing homes; (3) a greater ability and opportunity to retain and prolong an independent living style; (4) an improvement in health condition; and (5) a better sense of subjective well-being. The first experiment took place in The Hague and it emphasized the integration between sheltered housing and institutional services. The second was conducted in Enschede, and it combined sheltered housing with an extra infusion of social services and nursing care. As reported by Coolen et al. (1993) the evaluation of both experiments revealed very modest, almost negligible effects and they were confined, for the most part, to the residents' subjective sense of well-being. There was no reduction in the use of formal services or a more extensive use of the informal system of care.

The risk and need for intensive, skilled nursing home care cannot be averted but the Netherlands and Norway have been experimenting with temporary admissions and monitored discharges. Coolen et al. (1993) added, in the case of the Netherlands, that users tend to fall in two categories: (1) elderly dischargees from acute care hospitalization who lack viable support systems to assist them during their convalescence and recovery; and (2) chronically impaired elderly who cannot manage alone but whose informal carers are themselves temporarily incapacitated and in need of respite. Monk and Cox (1991) observed, in the Norwegian case, that some municipalities regularly bring frail elderly persons for short-term intensive care and subsequently return them to their homes in the community. This alternate sequence typically consists of one week in the nursing home for every three in their regular domiciles but there is no fixed pattern. The infusion of intensive services in question is meant to delay as much as possible the risk of permanent institutionalization.

Sweden has similarly attempted to bridge the dichotomy between institutional and community home care by advancing the "service house" concept as a social model of congregate, independent living where residents may receive home care services, according to individual need.

More specifically, service houses are owned and operated by the country's 282 municipal governments. A typical service house is a multistory complex of about 40 to 100 apartments, ranging from studios to three rooms with kitchen and bathroom. The building includes a cafeteria as well as activity and recreation rooms which are also open to other seniors from the adjacent community. The service house thus doubles as a multiservice center and even as a day and respite center for the neighborhood-at-large. Home help and home care services are available to each resident according to need but they are requisitioned from outside municipal and county agencies. These services are not an integral part of the residential facility and do not fall within the purview of its administration.

"Service houses" are meant to be a choice alternative to the more medicalized forms of institutional care. Relatives and discharge staff in hospitals point, however, to the fact that most "service house" residents are very old, dependent, confused and incapable of making appropriate personal decisions. They add that the needs of these residents often exceed the range of services available on the premises. Relatives, in particular, voice their disappointment over the lack of more custodial and personal care services. They would prefer that the "service house" become a full-fledged nursing home, as they find the distinction between them artificial or, in any event, not very convincing.

Service providers claimed, in turn, that a service strategy centered exclusively on both "service houses" and home care rests on an idyllic but false vision of the aging process (Monk and Cox, 1991). The assumption that most, if not all, older persons can be kept indefinitely in the community is not borne out by demographic forecasts which anticipate an older and sicker aged population. Nursing homes may well be, in the opinion of some of these respondents, the most humane solution for lonely and frail older persons. A nursing home provides round-the-clock attention and supervision, 24 hours a day or 168 hours a week. When at home, a frail person seldom receives more than 15 hours a week of home care services. In the absence of relatives or friends, they will be alone for the remaining 153 hours of the week. The objectives of "normalization" and "self-determination," as spelled out in the 1982 Social Services Act, are then of little relevance to many of these incapacitated and lonely persons. Many of these individuals would not mind a little less of the self-sufficiency and independence rhetoric in exchange for more company and more frequent care.

The above criticism leveled against the service houses was partially met in recent years with the design of a new variation of the "service" house, called "group dwellings" (*gruppboende*) for frail elderly, also targeted for dementia patients. These homes usually consist of smaller housing complexes with clusters of about eight persons sharing communal spaces but where each individual resides in his or her own room or small apartment. The staff of group houses is trained to provide more intensive care and round-the-clock supervision. Group houses are therefore a kind of hybrid that combines features of both institutional and community care but is regarded as the likely model and direction for the future (Johansson, 1993).

Denmark went even further with its recent Elderly Housing Act which reverses the traditional notion that potential residents have to fit into a range of static levels of care. It establishes, instead, the principle that services ought to adapt to the recipient, wherever he or she may reside. If a disabled older person needs intensive care, the nursing home should be brought to his or her regular habitual home, rather than the other way around, that is institutionalizing the person. As pointed out by Jamieson (1993), this virtual ubiquity and mobility of services may eventually end up doing away with the dichotomy between institutional and community-based home care. The flexibility intended in the new Danish legislation is not limited, however, to the environmental context where services are provided. It is also manifested in the operational continuity of the nurses and nurses aides, as well as, all other relevant personnel that follow their patients regardless whether they stay at home or are placed in an institutional setting.

The intent of creating flexible and adaptable environments, enriched with individually prescribed home care plans, would require a radical reorganization of the long-term care systems as presently constituted in the western industrial world. It may not be feasible without a highly centralized planning and administrative authority. This is just the opposite of the emerging trends toward organizational decentralization and the reaffirmation of welfare pluralism that are occurring in many of the western industrialized countries.

THE TREND TOWARD DECENTRALIZATION

Decentralized services, as found in England, Norway and Sweden, are intended to foster local and grass roots initiatives but they cannot preclude a certain degree of uniformity imposed from the top. Central governments fund a sizeable proportion of the local budgets and, in return, exact compliance with their own policy guidelines, which are aimed at ensuring a common denominator of operational procedures, as well as the universal adoption of minimum standards of care. The Audit Commission for Local Authorities in England and Wales, thus requires a clear statement of the aims of the service, a definition of the types of clients for whom coordination with other community services might be required, and guidelines on frequency and length of visits (Audit Commission, 1985).

More recently, the Griffiths parliamentary report (Her Majesty's Stationery Office, 1988) made cogent recommendations that strike a balance between the central government and the local authorities, as far as fiscal responsibility is concerned. It also reaffirmed that the mission of the public sector is to ensure the provision of services, without assuming the responsibility for the actual delivery of those services. It reasserted, to that effect, the participation of the private sector, through a purchase of services contractual mechanism.

Decentralization is not antithetical with coordination, nor should it be confounded with insularity. The Griffiths report consequently proposed attending to the clients' needs with services coordinated by a case manager, and also providing a single source of funding for community care, rather than the prevailing dual track of state and local funding.

Many of the recommendations contained in the Griffiths Report were subsequently incorporated in the government's White Paper, "Caring for People: Community Care in the Next Decade and Beyond" (Her Majesty's Stationery Office, 1989). The implementation of these recommendations started in April 1991, when each local authority was expected to have developed a plan for services, which would include some of the following key points: a needs assessment of the target population; objectives for community care in the next three years; assessment methods; the procedures by which services are to be purchased; training and case management provisions, and quality assurance systems. These plans are expected to complement those of the health and housing authorities and should also take into consideration the recommendations of other service providers and consumers.

The duties performed by the local social services were also expanded. In addition to the assessment of generic community needs, social services are also required to design individual service packages which strengthen the ability of older persons to live in the community. These packages are to incorporate individual preferences and build upon the assistance already provided by the informal support systems.

Case managers will play pivotal roles in assuring that individual needs are properly met, that resources are effectively managed, and that each person has an easily accessible and single point of entry into the service system. Additionally, the case manager will be responsible for monitoring the quality of care. Each local social service agency is expected to outline how they will use the case manager and how the manager will be linked to available resources.

Service delivery systems are expected to promote the development of domiciliary, day, and respite services, and needs assessments must take into account the roles of informal caregivers. Given that the implementation of the community care plans began in April, 1993, no data are yet available on the programs' effectiveness.

In addition to this national model for community care, local innovative programs in community care have also been initiated. An example is The Bexley Community Care Scheme which trains caregivers of the elderly to be their own case managers. Thus, the social workers provide information and assist the caregivers in finding additional benefits and in locating services and other persons who may help with the caregiving tasks. The social workers are involved only as consultants and enablers. The emphasis is on empowering the family and not in creating dependency.

In the case of Norway, the decentralization model also leaves the pragmatics of service delivery to the municipal authorities while the central government is circumscribed to defining desirable baseline or quality standards. The local governments, however, are not legally required to adopt the norms in reference. The country may thus be characterized as a federation of 453 autonomous governments, some hardly exceeding a few hundred residents, but each devising its own system of services. In practical terms there is substantial convergence among them. The local authorities abide, for the most part, with the central government's guidelines and they borrow from each others experience for the sake of expedience and savings. Also, they do not have at hand, nor can they afford the technological expertise usually concentrated in larger and far more complex units of government. What results is a *de facto* and tacitly agreed upon standardization, but it is not imposed from above. Yet there are subtle forms of arm-twisting and carrot-and-stick inducements central governments resort to. This is especially the case for Sweden where municipalities wishing to qualify for block grants–which subsidize 33% of the social service budgets–have no option but to conform to the operational guidelines and quality standards instituted by the central government.

What are positive attributes of a "decentralized" model? It is often claimed that: (1) it fosters the search for more creative service solutions; (2) it enhances professional decision making at the local level and consequently makes services more responsive to local needs; (3) it facilitates a client-centered approach to services, one that circumvents the pitfalls of indiscriminate uniformity; and (4) it makes it possible for the consumer to exercise freedom of choice. None of these positive consequences would be attainable under a monopolistic, centralized system. Services are thus personalized and regionalized because what works in one community may not necessarily be best suited for another.

And yet, decentralization has not assured equity or equal access to services. For three years in the early 1980s, Oslo experimented with decentralization in four of the 25 districts in which it was ultimately divided. The evaluation revealed that needy low income persons hardly availed themselves of home care services. As is the case in other countries, the more educated and economically better-off aged and disabled were the ones who maximized and benefitted from the use of public services.

Decentralization, most specially when coupled with purchase of services in the private sector, elicits fears of noncompliance and overbureaucratization. In countries that have traditionally relied upon the public and the voluntary sectors, there are fewer regulations or licensing provisions for private agencies as those found in the United States, to cite an extreme example. There are concerns that both the drafting of such standards and their subsequent enforcement would spearhead the creation of a new administrative layer of government, bound to siphon away the budgetary resources normally allocated for the direct provision of services.

CONCLUSION

Notwithstanding the extensive experimentation with new formulas for the delivery of home care services, the proportion of needy older persons who manage to benefit from these services in Europe is rather low. Less than 1 percent of the elderly population of age 65 and older receives home care in Spain (Walker et al., 1993). Even in countries that made an unmistakable programmatic commitment to advance home care, the level of provision still falls below the prevailing demand and community expectations.

As summarily reviewed in this chapter, some of the new strategies underscore tailor-made approaches of the case management or case mediator variety. The gist is to identify individual needs and broker the provision of services in an open market made up of public and private agencies. The ultimate objective here is to achieve efficiency and cost containment but, at the same time, to give consumers freedom of choice and a greater measure of control over the help they receive. Other experiments attempt to narrow the chasm between institutional and community-based services by means of more flexible residential models.

There are a number of distinctive "code" words presiding over these innovative efforts: decentralization, empowerment, self-help, etc. And of course, the already alluded normalization and substitution. Bringing them to reality is not that easy when even countries with planned economies and a welfare state tradition have to contend with problems such as the fragmentation of legal responsibility for the provision of services, lack of coordination between the health and the social services sector, the debate whether home care services should constitute a basic entitlement free of premiums and copayments, or whether beneficiaries should be required to shoulder some of the inherent costs, the linkage between home care services and rehabilitation services, the high turnover rates among home care workers and their need for more adequate training, etc. Regardless of the level of sophistication and creativeness achieved by myriad service experiments, one thorny and puzzling issue remains, for the most part unresolved. We are referring to the connection and complementarity between the formal service system and the families and relatives of the service recipient. There is substantial ambiguity as to who does what, and some policymakers harbor the illusion that families are ultimately capable of taking over most or the entire set of caregiving responsibilities.

Only one country, to our knowledge, confronted its demographic and social realities and accepted the fact that the number of older persons living alone, with shrinking and often virtually nonexisting networks of children and relatives, is on the rise. Denmark reached the unambiguous conclusion that home or domiciliary care has then to step in and take the lead (Holstein and Holst, 1993). Danish policymakers no longer subscribe to the principle of "subsidiarity" according to which the smallest social unit, namely the family must play a central role, followed–in the case of inability or absence of such unit–by the voluntary sector and only as a last resort, by the public sector. No wonder the supply of home care in Denmark has reached enviable and unmatched levels of adequacy in the continent. It was a pragmatic decision, for the most part, not a philosophical one. Ultimately every society will have to confront its own gerontic destiny and make the proper choice.

REFERENCES

Audit Commission for Local Authorities in England and Wales. (1985). *Managing social services for the elderly more effectively*. London: Her Majesty's Stationery Office.

Baldock, J. and Evers, A. (1991). In Krann, R. et al. (Eds.), *Care for the elderly: Significant innovations in three European countries*. Frankfurt am Main: European Center for Social Welfare Policy and Research, Campus/Westwood.

Berg, S., Branch, L.G., Doyle, A.E. and Sundstrom, G. (1988). "Institutional and home-based long term care alternatives: The 1965-1985 Swedish experience." *The Gerontologist*, 28, 825-829.

Binstock, R.H. (1983). "The aged as scapegoats." *The Gerontologist*, 23, 136-143.

Coolen, J.A. (Ed.). (1993). *Changing care for the elderly in the Netherlands: Experiences and research findings from policy experiments.* Assen/Maastrich: Van Gorcum.

Evers, A. and Leichsenring, K. (1994). "Paying for informal care: An issue of growing importance." *Ageing International*, XXI, 29-40.

Goewie, R. (1988). *Gezinsverzorging, een alternatief voor het verzorginsehuis.* Gravenhage: NIMAWO.

Guillemard, A.M., and Frossar, M. (1993). "Risks and achievements in strengthening home care: The case of France." In Evers, A. and Van der Zanden, G.H. (Eds.), *Better care for dependent people living at home.* Bunnik, the Netherlands: Netherlands Institute of Gerontology.

Her Majesty's Stationery Office. (1988). *Community care: Agenda for action. A report to the Secretary of State for Social Services by Sir Roy Griffiths.* London: Her Majesty's Stationery Office.

Her Majesty's Stationery Office. (1989, November). *Caring for people: Community care in the next decade and beyond.* London: Her Majesty's Stationery Office.

Holstein, B., Holst, E., Due, P., and Almind, G. (1993). "Formal and informal care for the elderly: Lessons from Denmark." In Evers, A. and Van der Zanden, G.H. (Eds.), *Better care for dependent people living at home.* Bunnik, the Netherlands: Netherlands Institute of Gerontology.

Jamieson, A. (1993). "Care for elderly people living at home: A European perspective." In Evers, A. and Van der Zanden, G.H. (Eds.), *Better care for dependent people living at home.* Bunnik, the Netherlands: Netherlands Institute of Gerontology.

Johansson, L. (1993). "Promoting home-based elder care: Some Swedish experiences." *Journal of Cross Cultural Gerontology*, 8, 391-406.

Kastelein, M., Dijkstra, A., and Schouten, C.C. (1989). *Care of the elderly in the Netherlands: A review of policies and services 1950-1990.* Leiden, the Netherlands: Institute of Preventive Health Care.

Ministry of Welfare, Health and Cultural Affairs. (January 1991). *Ageing matters: Portrait and policy: Focus on the elderly 1990-1994.* Rijswijk, the Netherlands: MWHCA.

Monk, A., and Cox, C. (1991). *Home care for the elderly: An international perspective.* Westport, CT: Auburn House.

Pijl, M.A. (1991). *Some recent developments in care for the elderly in the Netherlands.* Gravenhage, The Netherlands: Nederlands Instituut voor Maatschappelijk Werk Onderzoek.

Statistics Sweden. (1993). Statistika meddelanden, Social hemtjanst 1992 (Home help services 1992).

Szebehely, M. (1993). *Facts from statistics, reported in Hemtjanst eller anhorigvard? Forandringar under 1980-talet.* Stockholm, Sweden: National Board of Health and Welfare.

Szebehely, M. and Eliasson, R. (1991). "Hemtjansten I Sverige: Myter och statis-tik." *Nordisk Socialt Arbeid*, 1, 15-31.

Thorslund, M. (1992). *Care for the elderly in Sweden: Fact sheet.* Stockholm: The Swedish Institute.

Walker, A. (1993). "Towards a European agenda in home care for older people: Convergencies and controversies." In Evers, A. and Van der Zanden, G.H. (Eds.), *Better care for dependent people living at home.* Bunnik, the Nether-lands: Netherlands Institute of Gerontology.

Index

AARP (American Association of
  Retired Persons),
  26,91,134-135,214
Abramson, J.S., 173
Acceptance, transfer and discharge
  of patients, 35-36
Access to information systems, 112
Accreditation, 51-52
Activities of Daily Living (ADLs),
  162,218,220t
Adelman, J., 125
Adey, M., 223
ADLs (activities of daily living),
  162,218,220t
Administration. *See also* Supervision
  of case management services,
  238-239
  COHME (Concerned
  Homemakers for the
  Elderly) paradigm, 191-211
Administration on Aging. *See* U.S.
  Administration on Aging
Administrative issues
  admissions criteria, 72-75
  client assessment and education,
  81-83
  health needs assessment, 69-72
  program management, 76
  reimbursement, 75-76
  staffing, 76-81
Admissions
  computer-based processing, 91-92
  criteria for, 72-74
Advance medical directives, 40
Advertising, 139,148-149. *See also*
  Marketing
Affect, 221-223,224t
Agostinelli, B., 221

AHA (American Heart Association),
  41
AICD (Automatic Implantable
  Cardioverter Defibrillator),
  84-86
Albaum, G., 141
Almind, G., 268
Alzheimer's disease,
  19,170-178,218-221,222t
AMA (American Medical
  Association), 32
  home care guidelines, 126
American Association of Retired
  Persons (AARP),
  26,91,134-135,214
American Heart Association (AHA),
  41
American Medical Association
  (AMA), 32
  home care guidelines, 126
American Society for Parenteral and
  Enteral Nutrition, 88
Amyotrophic lateral sclerosis,
  178-182
Anderson, M., 33,42
Andrus Foundation (AARP),
  134-135
Anger, 176
Ansak, M., 26
Applebaum, R.A.,
  121,122,235,236,240
Applegate, W., 229
Arato, A., 84,85
Aronson, M.K., 213,218,221,223
Arras, J.D., 33,81
Arrhythmias, 84-86
Artificial nutrition/hydration, 87-89

© 1995 by The Haworth Press, Inc. All rights reserved.

Medicare, 12-15. *See also*
    Medicare
Older Americans Act funds, 22
private insurance, 23-26
social service block grants,
    21-22
state-funded programs, 23
veterans' benefits, 22-23
legal/ethical issues
    family's role, 37-39
    legal liability, 32-37
    limitation of treatment, 39-41
    physical or chemical restraints,
        41-42
    proactive addressing of, 42-43
    regulatory framework, 31-32
Pollard, W.E., 218
Polster, E., 177
Polster, M., 177
Popovich, B., 215
Popovich scale, 215,215t
Positioning, market, 142
Post, S.G., 41
Practice innovations
case management
    administration of services,
        238-239
    background, 233-234
    caseload size, 240
    continuum of care, 234-235
    evaluation, 247
    evolution of long-term care,
        235-236
    functions, 241-244
    objectives of, 236-238
    private vs. publicly funded and
        not-for-profit, 245-246
    qualifications of case manager,
        239-240
    quality improvement, 246-247
    staffing, 244
clinical assessment
    background and historical
        development, 213-214

care plan developed from,
    226-227
conclusion, 228-229
cultural diversity and, 225-226
future of home assessment,
    227-228
measurement issues, 227
process of, 215-225
state of the art, 214-215
counseling
    amyotrophic lateral sclerosis,
        178-182
    conclusions, 182-185
    elder/child in Alzheimer's
        disease, 170-178
    frail elder case, 161-162
    general principles, 159-160
    source of case examples,
        160-161
    terminally ill elder, 162-170
supervision
    COHME (Concerned
        Homemakers for the
        Elderly) paradigm, 191-211
    difficulties of COHME
        paradigm, 209-210
    direct client/family services,
        198-202
    marketing/outreach and,
        196-197
    organizational structure and,
        193-196
    reporting/documentation,
        192-198
    training and consultation,
        202-209
Pratt, C.C., 38
Priddy, J.M., 163
Pringle, D.M., 172
Privacy, 113. *See also*
    Confidentiality
Private duty nursing under Medicaid,
    19-20

Private vs. publicly funded and
    not-for-profit case
    management, 245-246
Process evaluations, 119-121
Proctor, E., 166
Products liability, 34-35
Professional endorsements, 150-151
Program innovations
    evaluations and quality assurance
      formative evaluations, 118
      outcome or summative
        evaluations, 121-129
      process evaluations, 119-121
    high-technology services. *See*
      also Technological
      innovation
      administrative issues, 69-83
      background and development,
        67-69
      treatment issues, 83-92
    information systems
      definition and perspectives,
        96-98
      development of,
        101,107,107f-108f
      example criteria, 102f-106f
      features and expected benefits,
        100-101
      and health care reform,
        111-113
      issues related to, 107-111
      literature review, 98-100
    marketing
      background and historical
        development, 133-136
      components of program,
        138-140
      conclusions, 154-155
      importance, 136-138
      participatory stance on,
        151-154
      promotional strategies,
        145-151
      special challenges in home
        health, 141-144

specialized markets, 144-145
organizational alternatives. *See*
    also Organization
    Community Nursing
      Organizations, 63-64
    determinants of structure,
      50-53
    examples of models, 54-58
    integrated delivery for elderly,
      56-62
    Living at Home/Block Nurse
      Program, 62-63
    success factors, 53-54
Program of All-inclusive Care for the
    Elderly (PACE), 60-62
Promotional strategies, 145-151. *See*
    also Marketing
Prospective Payment System, 68-69.
    See also Medicare
Public Law 101-508, 40,236
Public relations, 139-140. *See also*
    Marketing
Puget Sound (WA) Group Health
    Cooperative, 56,57f

Qualifying criteria. *See also*
    Eligibility
    Medicaid, 16
    Medicare, 12-15
Quality assurance
    evaluations
      formative, 118
      outcome or summative,
        121-129
      process, 119-121
    information systems criteria, 105t
Quality improvement in case
    management, 246-247
Quality of life, 252-253
Quality of marketing materials,
    149-151
Qualls, S.H., 166
Quinn, Joan, 233-247
Quinn, T., 149

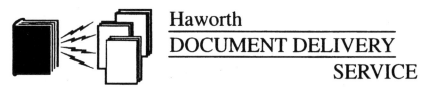

Haworth
DOCUMENT DELIVERY
SERVICE

This valuable service provides a single-article order form for any article from a Haworth journal.

- *Time Saving:* No running around from library to library to find a specific article.
- *Cost Effective:* All costs are kept down to a minimum.
- *Fast Delivery:* Choose from several options, including same-day FAX.
- *No Copyright Hassles:* You will be supplied by the original publisher.
- *Easy Payment:* Choose from several easy payment methods.

Open Accounts Welcome for ...
- Library Interlibrary Loan Departments
- Library Network/Consortia Wishing to Provide Single-Article Services
- Indexing/Abstracting Services with Single Article Provision Services
- Document Provision Brokers and Freelance Information Service Providers

---

MAIL or *FAX* THIS ENTIRE ORDER FORM TO:

Haworth Document Delivery Service
The Haworth Press, Inc.
10 Alice Street
Binghamton, NY 13904-1580

or **FAX:** 1-800-895-0582
or **CALL:** 1-800-342-9678
9am-5pm EST

PLEASE SEND ME PHOTOCOPIES OF THE FOLLOWING SINGLE ARTICLES:

1) Journal Title: _____
   Vol/Issue/Year:_____ Starting & Ending Pages:_____
   Article Title:_____
   _____

2) Journal Title: _____
   Vol/Issue/Year:_____ Starting & Ending Pages:_____
   Article Title:_____
   _____

3) Journal Title: _____
   Vol/Issue/Year:_____ Starting & Ending Pages:_____
   Article Title:_____
   _____

4) Journal Title: _____
   Vol/Issue/Year:_____ Starting & Ending Pages:_____
   Article Title:_____
   _____

(See other side for Costs and Payment Information)

COSTS: Please figure your cost to order quality copies of an article.

1. Set-up charge per article: $8.00
   ($8.00 × number of separate articles)   _____

2. Photocopying charge for each article:

   1-10 pages: $1.00   _____

   11-19 pages: $3.00   _____

   20-29 pages: $5.00   _____

   30+ pages: $2.00/10 pages   _____

3. Flexicover (optional): $2.00/article   _____

4. Postage & Handling: US: $1.00 for the first article/
   $.50 each additional article   _____

   Federal Express: $25.00   _____

   Outside US: $2.00 for first article/
   $.50 each additional article_____

5. Same-day FAX service: $.35 per page   _____

GRAND TOTAL: _____

METHOD OF PAYMENT: (please check one)

❑ Check enclosed   ❑ Please ship and bill. PO # _____
   (sorry we can ship and bill to bookstores only! All others must pre-pay)

❑ Charge to my credit card: ❑ Visa; ❑ MasterCard; ❑ Discover;
   ❑ American Express;

Account Number:_____ Expiration date:_____

Signature: ✗_____

Name: _____ Institution: _____

Address: _____

_____

City: _____ State:_____ Zip:_____

Phone Number: _____ FAX Number: _____

MAIL or *FAX* THIS ENTIRE ORDER FORM TO:

Haworth Document Delivery Service	**or FAX:** 1-800-895-0582
The Haworth Press, Inc.	**or CALL:** 1-800-342-9678
10 Alice Street	9am-5pm EST)
Binghamton, NY 13904-1580	